P9-CDB-508

# SAFE PATIENTS, SMART HOSPITALS

PETER PRONOVOST, M.D., PH.D., is a professor in the Department of Anesthesiology and the medical director of the Center for Innovation in Quality Patient Care and the Quality and Safety Research Group at Johns Hopkins University School of Medicine. Named one of *Time* magazine's "Most Influential People" in 2008, Dr. Pronovost was also the recipient of a MacArthur "genius" grant.

ERIC VOHR is a freelance author and editor, and teaches technical writing at Johns Hopkins University. His articles have appeared in the *Washington Post, Ski Magazine,* and the *Saturday Evening Post.* His media company, Vohr Communications (www.vohrcom.com), specializes in public relations, radio and video production, and professional writing.

---

"Both riveting and important . . . *Safe Patients, Smart Hospitals* gives an excellent overview of changes in hospital practice, which, when instituted, profoundly affect rates of serious medical complications and death. A pioneer in the field of patient safety, [Peter Pronovost] has radically altered how modern medicine is practiced."
—Kay Redfield Jamison, Ph.D., author of *An Unquiet Mind* and *Nothing Was the Same*

"No one in America has thought more—and done more—about patient safety than Dr. Pronovost. *Safe Patients, Smart Hospitals* is the right prescription for American health care."
—Sherrod Brown, United States senator (Ohio)

"Dr. Pronovost and Mr. Vohr offer a constructive and compelling case for patient safety and improving health care quality in the United States. Health providers and policy makers would benefit greatly from reading this book."
—Tom Daschle, former senator and author of *Critical: What We Can Do About the Health-Care Crisis*

"*Safe Patients, Smart Hospitals* reminds us how great change can be wrought by one person with the courage to do the right thing. Dr. Pronovost's account tells the thrilling story about how—not so long ago—sloppiness and medical arrogance made even the best American hospitals perilous places to spend the night. His remedy: something simple, elegant, convincing."
—Jean McGarry, professor at the Writing Seminars at Johns Hopkins University, and author of seven books of fiction

"A riveting account right from the first page . . . *Safe Patients, Smart Hospitals* is a must-read for everyone in health care, including consumers. The authors have covered particularly well the perspectives and challenges of nurses in keeping patients safe. The book is a 'good read' for us all."
—Linda H. Aiken, Ph.D., The Claire M. Fagin Leadership Professor of Nursing and Professor of Sociology, Director of the Center for Health Outcomes and Policy Research, University of Pennsylvania

# Safe Patients, Smart Hospitals

HOW ONE DOCTOR'S CHECKLIST
CAN HELP US CHANGE HEALTH CARE
FROM THE INSIDE OUT

## Peter Pronovost, M.D., Ph.D.,
### and
## Eric Vohr

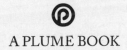

A PLUME BOOK

PLUME
Published by Penguin Group
Penguin Group (USA) Inc., 375 Hudson Street, New York, New York 10014, U.S.A. • Penguin Group
(Canada), 90 Eglinton Avenue East, Suite 700, Toronto, Ontario, Canada M4P 2Y3 (a division of Pearson
Penguin Canada Inc.) • Penguin Books Ltd., 80 Strand, London WC2R 0RL, England • Penguin Ireland, 25
St. Stephen's Green, Dublin 2, Ireland (a division of Penguin Books Ltd.) • Penguin Group (Australia), 250
Camberwell Road, Camberwell, Victoria 3124, Australia (a division of Pearson Australia Group Pty.
Ltd.) • Penguin Books India Pvt. Ltd., 11 Community Centre, Panchsheel Park, New Delhi – 110 017, India •
Penguin Books (NZ), 67 Apollo Drive, Rosedale, North Shore 0632, New Zealand (a division of Pearson New
Zealand Ltd.) • Penguin Books (South Africa) (Pty.) Ltd., 24 Sturdee Avenue, Rosebank, Johannesburg 2196,
South Africa

Penguin Books Ltd., Registered Offices: 80 Strand, London WC2R 0RL, England

Published by Plume, a member of Penguin Group (USA) Inc. Previously published in Hudson Street
Press edition.

First Plume Printing, February 2011
10  9  8  7  6  5  4  3  2  1

Ⓟ  REGISTERED TRADEMARK—MARCA REGISTRADA

The Library of Congress has catalogued the Hudson Street Press edition as follows:

Pronovost, Peter J.
    Safe patients, smart hospitals : how one doctor's checklist can help us change
healthcare from the inside out / Peter Pronovost and Eric Vohr.
    p. cm.
    ISBN 978-1-59463-064-4 (hc.)
    ISBN 978-0-452-29686-2 (pbk.)
    1. Medical errors—Prevention.   2. Hospitals—Safety measures.   3. Lists.   I. Vohr,
Eric.   II. Title.
    R729.8.P76 2010
    610.28'9—dc22          2009051768

Printed in the United States of America
Set in Adobe Caslon Pro with Candida • Original hardcover design by Daniel Lagin

PUBLISHER'S NOTE
Penguin is committed to publishing works of quality and integrity. In that spirit, we are proud to offer this
book to our readers. However, the story, the experiences, and the words are the authors' alone. We would
like to state that although the majority of this book takes place at Johns Hopkins, the events described
can and do occur at other medical centers, clinics, and hospitals. Every effort has been made to ensure
that the information contained in this book is complete and accurate. However, neither the publisher nor
the authors are engaged in rendering professional advice or services to the individual reader. The ideas,
procedures, and suggestions contained in this book are not intended as a substitute for consulting with
your physician. All matters regarding your health require medical supervision. Neither the authors nor
the publisher shall be liable or responsible for any loss or damage allegedly arising from any information
or suggestion in this book.

*This book is dedicated to my father. —P. P.*

# Introduction

On a cool January evening in 2001, the King family sat down to eat in a cluttered room that served as dining room, kitchen, living room, and playroom. The family of six had recently moved into a green shingled, ramshackle farmhouse, perched on a grassy hill in the country outside of Baltimore, and were having it renovated. Many of the rooms had been gutted and stacks of two-by-fours and sheets of plywood cluttered the hallways.

Dinner was takeout Thai food, since there wasn't much of a kitchen. Sorrel King opened a bottle of wine to celebrate the arrival of her mother, who had driven up from Virginia to see the new house. Sorrel's youngest, eighteen-month-old Josie, danced to the Barney song "I Love You" that played on her little music cube. Her three older children, Jack, six, Relly, five, and Eva, three, slipped upstairs to watch their favorite cartoon, *Rugrats*.

Sorrel, her husband, Tony, and Sorrel's mother, whom everybody called "Big Rel," talked about the work they had left to do on the house as they poured wine and dished out pad Thai and curried chicken on paper plates. And then Sorrel suddenly became aware that the Barney song had stopped.

"Where's Josie?" she asked, concerned that her youngest had slipped out of sight. Before she got an answer, a terrified scream shook the old wooden house.

Earlier that evening, Big Rel had entertained the kids while she took a bubble bath in an upstairs bathroom the Kings never used. The bathroom had an old cast-iron tub that fascinated the precocious young Josie. Big Rel let the curious infant float her toy airplane on the piles of white bubbles that overflowed onto the floor. While the Kings were preparing to eat, Josie had followed her siblings upstairs and made a beeline for that old tub.

Responding to her daughter's screams, Sorrel bolted upstairs and found Josie standing in the bathroom wailing hysterically, her arms sticking out from her sides, her pink onesie soaking wet. Sorrel yelled down to Tony to call 911 and frantically undressed the screaming child. The pajamas were hot to the touch, especially the rubber parts on her feet. When she exposed Josie's skin it was red and raw—a stark contrast to the child's bright blue eyes and wild locks of soft blonde hair. Sorrel looked in the tub: it was partially filled with water and Josie's toy plane was floating innocently on the surface. She touched the water; it was scalding hot.

Josie must have wanted to see her plane float in the tub again and had turned on the faucet. Unfortunately, she had turned on the one with *H* written on it. Sorrel later learned that the water heater in that old house was broken, which made the water that hit Josie's tender young skin near boiling temperature.

When the medics arrived they carefully wrapped Josie's burned arms and legs in white gauze and placed her in the back of the ambulance. Josie had received second-degree burns on 60 percent of her body—a critical injury for anyone, but especially bad for a child at her young age. Sorrel rode along in the ambulance to the hospital, her eyes fixed on her suffering child. She kept telling herself, "Josie is going to be okay; she's going to be okay."

When Josie arrived at the burn unit at Johns Hopkins Bayview Medical Center, they had difficulty getting an IV into the child because of her burns, so she was transferred to the pediatric intensive care unit (PICU) at Johns Hopkins Children's Center—the place best equipped to treat the most critically ill children.

Second-degree burns destroy the skin's ability to control temperature and fluids. This is especially serious for children who have less skin for their body mass than adults. Second-degree burns are also more painful than third-degree burns, which are technically worse. Second-degree burns kill the skin, but don't go deep enough to kill the nerve roots, so the patient can still feel. The excessive pain associated with second-degree burns can cause major physiological problems like increased heart rate and high blood pressure.

One of the doctors' first priorities was to make sure Josie was getting intravenous fluids, so they placed IVs in her neck, wrist, and inner thigh. A few days later in the operating room, doctors would replace these lines with a central line catheter, a semipermanent tube that ran through the blood vessels to a place just outside the little girl's heart so doctors could administer fluids, nutrients, and medication more efficiently and also monitor heart function.

As their injured child lay in the PICU hooked up to a myriad of complex machines with a breathing tube in her throat, Sorrel and Tony sat anxiously by her bedside—their world had stopped.

The Kings had moved to Baltimore in 1999 from Richmond, Virginia. Tony, thirty-four, an investment banker at Wachovia, had transferred to Baltimore to open a new trading desk. Sorrel, also thirty-four, was taking time off from a successful career designing women's clothing to be a stay-at-home mom.

The Kings were a typical large, happy, young family—toys on the floor, kids running around, and a big, happy, smelly dog adding to the confusion. As the youngest in the family, Josie assumed a position of privilege. She had just learned to say "I wuv you, I wuv you" and she loved her sisters and brother dearly. Most of all, she adored her parents and was the first to make it clear that she was their number-one priority.

Lying motionless in a tiny hospital bed at Hopkins, she was just that. Every bit of her parents' hearts and souls were focused on this little girl who was struggling to stay alive. The hospital became Sorrel's new home. Often accompanied by her husband and her younger sister, Margaret, who lived in Washington, D.C., Sorrel would seldom leave her little girl's side.

Sorrel offered to help the staff whenever she could, and she soon became fond of the people entrusted with Josie's care. She brought them coffee and muffins and tried her best not to interfere with their work.

"I thought they were brilliant and I was so thankful I was at Hopkins with them taking care of Josie. Thank God," says Sorrel. "I was moved by everything I saw. I was just in awe the entire time I was there in the PICU—the doctors, the nurses—I mean they were amazing. I would go down and get my coffee and my muffins and see these posters on the walls of the hospital—magazine covers from *U.S. News and World Report* listing Johns Hopkins as the number one hospital in the United States. I thought, I am so lucky that I am at Hopkins."

During her first days in the hospital, doctors and nurses worked hard to help Josie heal and recover. In the operating room, surgeons transplanted skin from the parts of Josie's body that were not burned. What skin grafts the doctors could not get from Josie, they got from a donor. They removed dead tissue, changed her sterile dressings regularly to protect against infection, and implanted a "pain pump" that would safely deliver powerful narcotics to ease Josie's suffering.

When she wasn't by Josie's side, Sorrel slept on a cot in a special room the Children's Center keeps for parents who have very ill children. The doctors and nurses tried to convince Sorrel to go home and get proper rest, but she wanted to stay close to her little girl. "I wanted to take care of Josie because she was my baby. I wanted to be there," says Sorrel.

In the room where she slept, each of the cots had a curtain drawn around it for privacy. She was often the last one in and the first one out and never met any of the others who were staying there. However, in the corner of the room there was a journal that contained the words of parents who had passed through this place. One night Sorrel picked up the journal and started reading.

"I remember reading these stories, some in foreign languages. The ones I could understand told stories of their children with sickle-cell anemia and children with cancer. These parents traveled from all over the world to come to Hopkins. I remember thinking that these people have real problems, my story doesn't belong in here, Josie is going home in a few days," recalls Sorrel.

While the doctors and nurses treated Josie, Sorrel pored over books about burns and regularly discussed procedures with the doctors. Sorrel only briefly left the hospital in order to spend time with her other children. To help out, her mother stayed in Baltimore and looked after the house and kids during Sorrel's long absences.

Eventually, Josie's condition began to improve. Her breathing tube was removed and her burns began to heal. The child moved to solid food.

"She had the feeding tube and now she was eating Jell-O, trying to use a fork; it was so exciting just to see her eat. It made me so happy to see Josie start to look normal again," says Sorrel. Then the best news of all came: the doctors told her she might be able to bring her daughter home in as little as ten days.

"It was the happiest day of my life when I knew she was coming home," says Sorrel.

Just before Valentine's Day, Josie was well enough to be moved out of the PICU and down to the intermediate care unit. To prepare Josie for her upcoming trip home, doctors removed her pain pump and started her on methadone, a drug that helps patients avoid the effects of withdrawal from pain medication.

Josie's brothers and sisters were busy preparing for her homecoming. They inflated colored balloons and made cards. Sorrel began making plans to redecorate Josie's room.

"I wanted her to come home to a big girl's room," Sorrel recalled thinking at the time.

Sorrel also began preparation for a party to honor all those who had helped her through this crisis, including the doctors and nurses who were taking such good care of her little girl.

And then things started to go wrong.

Josie developed a fever and started vomiting regularly. On February 18, Josie's temperature was 102. On February 19, tests confirmed a bacterial infection in her blood that had come from her central line catheter, a type of infection called a central line–associated bloodstream infection. Doctors removed the catheter and started administering oral antibiotics. Though these infections are usually treated with intravenous antibiotics, Josie was started on oral antibiotics because her scarring made it difficult to get an intravenous line into her skin. If the doctors thought Josie would be staying with them longer, they probably would have worked harder to establish an IV line, but many in the care team were convinced this child would soon be on her way home.

Josie continued to vomit and developed diarrhea—common reactions to antibiotics, which kill many of the helpful bacteria that aid in food digestion. Without a central or intravenous line supplying liquids to her body, Josie's diarrhea and vomiting continued to deplete her body of fluids.

Sorrel noticed that her daughter kept crying and reaching out to anyone who came near her with a drink. Sorrel says she told nurses she thought Josie was dehydrated. But the nurses would not let her give her daughter water or juice, only ice chips. According to Sorrel, the nurses said that because of Josie's diarrhea and vomiting they were afraid fluids might upset her stomach and make her worse. At Sorrel's request, doctors checked Josie's heart and respiratory rates, blood pressure, temperature, and weight. They also reviewed her "ins" and "outs"—food and drink, as well as urine and stool and any vomit.

"They told me that her vitals were fine," says Sorrel. "I said, 'She is really thirsty—can we hook her up to an IV?' They said, 'She is fine. Kids look like this when they have been in the hospital for a long time.'"

Sorrel was worried her daughter's condition was deteriorating and wasn't convinced the doctors and nurses were seeing what she was seeing. Parents can offer valuable insights into a child's condition that is often not appropriately valued by members of the care team. In this case Sorrel was right. The oral antibiotics were killing helpful bacteria in Josie's digestive system. As a result, the weakened Josie had developed a secondary infection in her intestines. That meant that she was now fighting two infections—one from the central line and one from her intestines. Josie was septic, a serious condition that can have lethal consequences.

To further complicate matters, these two infections were adding to the dehydrating effects of the vomiting and diarrhea. Infections like these cause fluid to literally leak out of blood vessels into surrounding tissue, effectively lowering the amount of fluid in the circulatory system. Blood pressure can drop and bad things can start to happen. The brain can shut down, organs can die, and the heart can stop pumping.

This type of dehydration can be challenging for clinicians to quickly detect because it does not show up in the two standard tests that indicate fluid loss—weight and the monitoring of "ins" and "outs." Her weight would not initially reflect fluid loss due to the central line infection because her body was not technically losing fluids, but rather redistributing them. Similarly, her "ins" and "outs" would only reflect what she was consuming and discharging, not what was being stored in tissue. For an adult, this might not be as serious since a fully grown body has such a large volume of blood. But an infant has a much smaller circulatory system, and small, undetected changes in blood volume can have devastating effects.

"That evening I gave her a bath. When she was naked in the bathtub she seemed very thin, and she kept sucking on the washcloth trying to drink," says Sorrel. "I put her in bed and her eyes kind of rolled back in her head. I told the nurses, we have to get a doctor in here, something is not right."

At this point some of the nurses said they also suspected that Josie was not doing well. Despite Josie's stable vital statistics, instinct and experience told them this child was potentially in danger. The nurses said they tried to communicate these concerns to the surgeons but didn't feel their concerns were taken seriously.

The nurses and the child's mother were likely the ones who first noticed Josie's deteriorating condition because they spent the most time with the child. The surgeons, who ultimately made the final decisions regarding Josie's care, were much less often at the bedside. That's the way many hospitals are structured. Surgeons spend a lot of time in the operating room. This is what they are trained to do; they need to develop their skills and treat patients. As a result they must depend more heavily on numbers and charts to judge a patient's condition and often can only manage a couple of brief visits a day. And as we learned with Josie, the numbers are sometimes deceiving. Nurses and, often, family members have the most comprehensive, day-to-day, hour-by-hour knowledge of a patient's every changing condition. And that was especially significant in Josie's case. This little girl's condition changed rapidly in a short amount of time.

The nurses said they tried to voice their concerns up the chain of command but no action was taken. The way communication was organized at Hopkins, and most hospitals during that time, did not make this easy. Nurses would have to talk to residents, who then passed the message on to chief residents or fellows, who then would talk to the attending surgeons. It is common for the opinion of lower levels of the hierarchy to be discounted and often ignored by higher-ups. Every player along the way could theoretically decide the message was not significant enough to pass up, and it would die right there. Furthermore, surgeons are often busy in the operating room and unavailable or hard to reach, which only complicates this communication even more. If someone jumps rank or seeks approval from another surgeon outside of the chain or in any way circumvents this hierarchy, the penalty is often public humiliation and reprimand. In these ways a critical message can get tangled and lost in a complex archaic culture that puts patients at risk.

The next morning Sorrel got coffee and muffins for the nurses and headed up to the unit. When she got in the room she was shocked at how bad Josie appeared.

"Josie was lethargic and unresponsive; she was very pale and looked almost unconscious. She was a lot worse than the night before," says Sorrel. "I went up the hallway and screamed for help. Up to this point I tried to be low maintenance. I didn't want to ask too many questions; I did not want to be in anyone's way; I brought muffins and coffee for the nurses. Now I was screaming for help. I said, 'Docs, you have to come.' They were doing their rounds. They said, 'We'll be there in a little bit, Mom (they called me 'Mom!') we have some other patients we need to see; they were before you.' I said, 'No, you've got to come now.' And then they came."

According to Sorrel this was the first time she felt the doctors realized Josie was not doing very well. Worried that her condition might be related to the methadone treatments, the doctors gave her Narcan—a powerful drug that counteracted the effects of methadone. Josie almost immediately perked up, so the doctors canceled the methadone treatments.

While this might make it seem that methadone was the problem, Josie's condition was much more complicated than that. Severe dehydration due to the infections and septic shock were more likely the underlying reasons why Josie had deteriorated, not methadone. During extreme cases of dehydration, blood vessels constrict to increase blood pressure so blood can reach the brain. Methadone, and sepsis, relax these blood vessels and blood pressure drops—which could have contributed to Josie's lethargic behavior. The Narcan corrected this drop in blood pressure, but did not address the core issue—Josie's infections and resulting dehydration.

At Sorrel's request, the doctors let Josie drink. She greedily consumed almost a liter of fluids, which made Sorrel happy. She, like others, believed the methadone was the problem. It seemed obvious: the Narcan had transformed Josie from a nearly unconscious, lethargic infant to an alert, responsive, healthy-looking child.

"She was doing great," says Sorrel. "She drank the water; she didn't throw up. I thought, phew, she is going to be okay."

Later that morning, a new pain specialist, who was also a pediatrician and anesthesiologist, came on service. She said when she first saw Josie she was not fully convinced that methadone was the problem. She believed Josie was very sick with sepsis and the only reason her vital statistics were strong was because her body was compensating. This is what people do when they are sick—the body does whatever is necessary to stay alive. But the pain specialist said she knew Josie couldn't keep this up for long and wanted to move Josie back to the PICU. However, the hierarchal structure did not give her the power to make this decision. She said she told one of the surgeons that she thought Josie was going to crash and should be moved to the PICU. But, according to the pain specialist, the surgeon told her Josie looked better than ever and Josie was not moved to the PICU.

There is some dispute as to what conversations actually took place between team members as Josie started to get worse. Both the nurses and the pediatric pain specialist say they talked to the residents about their concerns about Josie and feel their concerns were ignored. The surgical attending says he was never notified of these concerns. However, one thing seems crystal clear: communication between these teams was poor. And as a result, Josie's care most likely suffered.

The pain specialist had another concern. By taking Josie suddenly off of her methadone and giving her Narcan, this doctor was convinced the little girl would start to experience severe withdrawal symptoms, which would only further compromise her fragile condition. She got approval from one of the surgeons to give Josie methadone again, but half of the normal dose.

Sorrel was in the room with one of the nurses, rubbing bacitracin ointment on Josie's hands and feet to fight infection. A second nurse appeared, carrying a plastic syringe used to administer medications orally. Sorrel asked the second nurse what she was doing. The nurse told her that she was giving Josie methadone—as ordered.

"I was thinking, should I knock the methadone out of her hand and scream for help?" says Sorrel.

But she did not follow this instinct. Instead she told herself that she was in the best hospital in the country and the doctors must have changed the order because they knew what was best for Josie.

"I thought, Josie must need this medication. It's really important that she gets it so she can get better. They know her better than I do," recalls Sorrel.

The nurse who was helping Sorrel rub ointment on her daughter's feet said, "Oh, look, a crocodile tear." Josie had one little tear running down her cheek. As Sorrel wiped it away she thought it strange. In the two weeks she had been at Hopkins, Josie had never cried or shed a tear. Then Sorrel watched in horror as Josie's eyes rolled back into her head. Her heart had stopped beating.

"I was shaking her and then the nurses were pushing buttons, then doctors and a lot of people came into the room with trays, tables, and carts and things and then they were doing all this stuff, and one of them said, 'What the hell happened here?'"

Josie wasn't breathing and she had no pulse. Sorrel was whisked into the hall and the team started chest compressions. Josie vomited into her oxygen mask, and one of the clinicians inserted a breathing tube.

"I am out there in the hall looking into the room at all these doctors surrounding Josie's bed. I couldn't see Josie. I was in shock, I knew, I couldn't do anything; they were all around her. I just wanted them to do their thing. And then they put me in a room with a chaplain and no windows," recalls Sorrel.

The doctors, realizing the patient was severely dehydrated, struggled to get an IV into Josie's arm or leg veins but failed because of the scarring from her burns. As a last resort, they inserted a needle into the marrow of a bone in her leg in a futile attempt to hydrate the poor dying girl. The first resuscitation attempts failed and more doctors arrived; someone managed to get an IV into Josie's femoral vein. Fifteen minutes passed, but Josie still had no pulse.

Just as they were about to let her go, Josie's heart started beating again.

"I don't know how much time went by. They eventually took me up the back steps to the PICU. I walked in, the doctors were standing around her bed; she was all hooked up with things coming out of every part of her body. Her leg was black and blue; there was blood and stuff; she looked horrible. But I said, 'This is okay, this is going to be fine, you guys did this to her, I know you can fix her, you're the best in the world.' I said, 'Everything is okay, don't worry about it, you did this, you can fix her, I know you can, I don't care what it costs, I don't care what it takes, we will spend the money, we will get whatever transplant you need, tell us what organ, we'll make it happen, we'll get it, we will do whatever we can do, anything.' The doctors could hardly look at me. They said, 'We need to pray.'"

Sorrel's husband, Tony, had left on a business trip and his plane had just touched down in California. When he heard the news,

Tony immediately got on a flight back to Baltimore. The next morning the neurologists examined Josie; they wouldn't let Sorrel or Tony stay in the room, so the anxious parents waited in the hall with the rest of the family.

"When the doctors had finished, they came out and said Josie was brain-dead. Although her heart was still beating, she had no brain stem function. I said, 'There will be a miracle. I was just in the waiting room with a mother and her daughter and they had a miracle,'" recalls Sorrel. But there was no miracle, Josie was gone.

Even though it appeared as though the methadone made Josie's heart stop, the hospital later concluded Josie died because of dehydration and sepsis due primarily to her central line infection and an intestinal infection. Central line infections are very common when a patient has a central line catheter for a long time or one is inserted in nonsterile conditions. These infections kill between thirty thousand and sixty thousand people in the United States each year and are largely preventable.

In addition, the hospital concluded that poor communication between care team members also contributed to Josie's death. Specifically, key members of the team missed signs that Josie condition was deteriorating and did not take proper action, which would have been to get Josie to intensive care and treat her dehydration with intravenous fluids. Josie's heart stopped because her body ran out of reserves to keep compensating. She was severely dehydrated, her veins collapsed, and there just wasn't enough blood pressure to keep her heart beating.

In the bigger picture, however, what really killed Josie was an archaic culture that disabled the care team so they did not recognize and act on the obvious signs that Josie was dehydrated. Sorrel, and some of the nurses and physicians, suspected that Josie was in danger. But these concerns were perhaps not properly respected or heeded and as a result not enough action was taken.

Even more distressing is that we now know these infections are almost universally preventable. Placing central lines without using proper barrier precautions, or not managing central lines properly after they are in place, is the most common cause of these infections.

On February 22, a family friend and minister, Thomas G. Speers, christened Josie while her mother and father stood by in shock and disbelief. Their precious daughter, hooked up to life support, just stared up at the ceiling, her eyes fixed and vacant. Sorrel brought Josie's siblings, Jack, Relly, and Eva, to say good-bye, but the children were confused about what was happening and did not want to kiss their sister good-bye.

After the children left the room, Josie's family stood around the small dying child hooked up to a myriad of bleeping, buzzing machines. Speers read from the Bible as doctors placed the near-lifeless child into her parents' arms.

"We held her and they switched off the machines. We held her and we held her. Her heart was still beating and the doctor came up and put the stethoscope on her heart and then he nodded, which meant her heart had stopped, she was dead," recalls Sorrel.

The grief-stricken parents each held their precious child for the last time, rocking her and singing to her through their tears as light flakes of snow softly fell outside the window.

Josie King's death had a significant impact on Johns Hopkins. Like all hospitals, Hopkins was no stranger to medical errors. However, the senseless death of this eighteen-month-old child affected nurses, physicians, and administrators at all levels. Perhaps it was her tender young age, or the bonds that had formed between doctors, nurses, and the King family during that agonizing month before she died. Or perhaps this error shined a spotlight on communication and teamwork failures that clearly harm patients; perhaps the time had come for a change.

# Chapter 1

===

Since 1955, the average life expectancy in the United States has increased from sixty-nine to seventy-eight years. Thanks to American medical research, many terminal cancers are now curable, AIDS has become a manageable chronic illness, and some patients can live with the once universally fatal cardiovascular disease. The United States is more productive in biomedical research than the entire European Union combined. And the world continues to look toward the United States for major breakthroughs in medicine.

Yet with all this knowledge and science at their disposal, physicians only provide about half of the known recommended treatments to the millions of adults and children who seek medical care in the United States annually. Even more disturbing, it is estimated that hundreds of thousands of patients will die each year as a result of a medical error. Well-intentioned doctors leave instruments in patients, overdose children with medications, and operate on the wrong side of the body.

Anyone who has felt dissatisfied with the quality or safety of medical care knows that medicine is failing to consistently perform its number-one priority: healing patients. Trust and faith in doctors is gradually eroding, forcing people to assume a larger role in their own health care. Those seeking medical care often search extensively for the best doctor, gather multiple opinions, scan the Web for medical advice and diagnoses, and/or bring along a spouse or loved one to sit by their bedside to ensure that they receive the best possible care. All of this while the United States spends roughly eight thousand dollars per person on health care, nearly twice as much as any other developed nation.

And although it is important that patients are well educated about the care they receive, this approach is an inefficient way to gain access to good health care. It is also no guarantee that they will be safe from harm. Sorrel King practically lived at the hospital and did extensive research on Josie's illness and care. But in the end, it didn't matter. Josie still fell victim to hospital errors and died likely as a result of these errors.

In 1999 the Institute of Medicine came out with an influential report on medical errors, "To Err Is Human," that shined a spotlight on the "hidden" problem of patient safety. Based on analysis of a number of independent studies, it concluded that between forty-four thousand and ninety-eight thousand people die each year in the United States as a result of preventable medical errors. And this number does not likely include diagnostic errors, infections, and patients who die from not receiving recommended treatments.

It was in 1987, a decade before that report was issued, during my first year at Johns Hopkins University School of Medicine, that I first knew I would devote my career to improving patient safety. At that point, none of the top medical institutions, including Hopkins, offered a single course or program in this field. It was not even discussed. Yet I had decided this was what I wanted to do with my medical education. I felt I had little choice; the gears of fate had begun turning four years earlier when I experienced a tragedy that literally changed the course of my life.

It was May 1984 and I had just finished the last exam of my freshman year at Fairfield University in Connecticut. I was really more of a jock than an academic. I had been captain of the swim and lacrosse teams in high school and joined the swim team at college. Although I found my academic studies relatively easy, I lacked maturity and discipline in my intellectual pursuits. Little did I know my world was about to change dramatically.

My parents had driven down to visit from our home in Waterbury an hour to the north and I ran across the quad to meet them. As soon as I got into the car, I knew something was wrong. Both of my parents had tears in their eyes. In a broken voice my father told me that he had cancer.

I listened, holding back tears and biting my lip. It seemed impossible to me that my father of forty-five, with whom I often went on runs, could have a potentially fatal disease. It transformed my sense of what was real, what was important. The adult world of responsibility, tragedy, and sorrow had come crashing into my sheltered and idyllic college life. As they explained the diagnosis and treatment and his chances of survival I said very little; I just sobbed. When they had finished I asked them if I could have a little time to myself; I left the car, changed into my running clothes, and went for a long run. I ran harder, faster, and longer than I would have if I were running a track meet; I wanted the physical pain to defeat the emotional pain; yet the emotional pain was more powerful and refused to yield.

As I doggedly placed one foot in front of the other, my head was filled with doubt, fear, and confusion. I knew a tremendous responsibility had just fallen on my shoulders—a responsibility to work hard in school, make something of my life, and add something good to the world. I wanted my parents, especially my dad, to be proud of me; perhaps my success would help them emotionally and physically.

During my college years, my dad was in and out of the hospital. The type of chemotherapy he was receiving literally ate away at his bones, so in addition to his cancer, he also needed hip replacement surgery. It was a very difficult and painful time in our lives and I spent every free moment I could at my father's side. When he went in for his hip surgery, my brothers, my friends, and I even joined him in his hospital room to watch the Chicago Bears defeat the New England Patriots in Super Bowl XX. When I wasn't with my family, I poured myself into my books. This tragedy had given me focus I previously lacked, a focus that made it possible for me to get into Johns Hopkins medical school.

In my first year at Hopkins we were told his diagnosis had changed from lymphoma to leukemia. The doctors said this was a particularly deadly form of cancer and there wasn't much they could do. Even though I knew little about medicine then, something didn't quite add up. I asked my parents if they would come and talk to one of the cancer specialists at Johns Hopkins.

After talking to an oncologist at Hopkins, it became clear to me that my father had been subject to a medical error. It was difficult to decipher because the doctor spoke in a code. Like most physicians he was probably cautious to judge another physician. At times, I likely speak the same language myself now, perhaps without even realizing it.

The Hopkins physician told my father, "Had you come in earlier, I would have offered you a bone marrow transplant. The cancer that you have is notoriously difficult to cure. Without catching it early and treating it with a transplant, the chance of survival is slim. Unfortunately, now it is too late, and you are beyond the stage that we could offer you this treatment. All we can suggest now is palliative care."

The doctor essentially told us that my father, at one time, could have been saved, but now he was most certainly going to die. I couldn't believe what I was hearing. My father was only forty-nine. You could barely tell he had cancer. He had soft smooth skin, thick brown wavy hair, and bright blue eyes that sparkled with life; it was hard to imagine he was going to die. The physician didn't use the word "mistake," and he never said that an error had occurred. Yet it was pretty clear to me this was what had happened.

My understanding of medicine was extremely limited at the time. I was essentially just like the millions of patients and family members who walk into hospitals across the country every day, either sick themselves or accompanying a sick loved one like my father. I did not fully understand the difference between leukemia and lymphoma; I did not understand what types of cancers could be treated with bone marrow transplants and which could not. And, like so many others, I wanted to believe these doctors had done all they could to save my father. I tried to tell myself that this was just the way things happen, the inevitability of life, but it didn't settle well with me. I was sure my father could have and should have received better care.

My father's condition continued to get worse and eventually he was hospitalized with severe pain and high calcium in his blood. Both the chemotherapy and the cancer had chewed away at his bone marrow, leaving his skeleton brittle. The smallest movements literally broke his bones, leaving him with multiple fractures in his vertebrae and hips.

Eager to be united again as a family during his last days, we arranged for home hospice care and had a hospital bed put in my parents' room. I took leave from school the summer after my third year of medical school, as did my brother, who was an intern at a hospital in Hartford, Connecticut. I vividly remember carrying my father's crumbling eighty-pound body up to his room. He was writhing in pain and had a look of immense suffering. He was getting morphine, but it was not enough to dull the agony.

The hospice care was woefully inadequate. One day when it was obvious he was in a lot of pain I spoke to the hospice nurses and asked if they could do something more to alleviate his suffering. She gave me a cold and detached response: "There is nothing we can do; your father has already received all the pain medicine he is going to get."

We never left my father alone. At night we would take turns sleeping in his room. I would lie in my parents' bed while my father slept in the adjacent hospital bed. He was in such agony he would moan and suffer continuously; it was torture to listen to him. One night he developed seizures, most likely due to the effects of the chemotherapy or an electrolyte abnormality. These seizures were terrifying to watch. His body and limbs shook violently; he lost control of his bowels and bladder. With his bones so brittle, these seizures also produced more fractures and more pain. Seizures are easily treated with common medicines like Valium, yet the hospice workers didn't have these drugs and were therefore incapable of treating them. My father was left to suffer unnecessarily.

Frustrated with the poor care my father was receiving, my brother and I took matters into our own hands. Since the hospice team would not supply my father with Valium, we would get it ourselves. So we drove down to the local hospital in our town where my brother had once worked as a medical student, explained the situation, and managed to get some Valium. As soon as we got home we treated my father. His seizures stopped and he was able to sleep through the night.

The next evening, at two a.m., I got up to see how he was doing and the nurse confronted me. I assumed she was going to challenge me for having independently procured Valium for my father. Instead she asked if my parents' big king-size bed where I was sleeping was lonely for just one person and wondered if I wanted some company. I couldn't believe my ears. With my father dying in the bed next to me, with my obvious dissatisfaction with her team's poor level of care, her only response was to proposition me? It was absurd and tragic. All I could ask myself was, is this the status of modern palliative care?

When my father finally passed away I returned to medical school to finish my studies. The experience had changed the way I viewed health care. My dad had suffered and died needlessly at the premature age of fifty thanks to medical errors and poor quality of care. In addition, my family and I also needlessly suffered. As a young doctor I vowed that, for my father and my family, I would do all that I could to improve the quality and safety of care delivered to patients. The health care system is capable of giving patients far better care. And patients deserve much more.

Many years later, I was giving a talk on my work in patient safety to physicians at Johns Hopkins. In the audience was a gastroenterologist named Dr. David Cromwell. I first met David when I was a medical student and he was a medical resident.

David approached me after the talk and said, "Peter, that was powerful. Those ideas could change health care. You should speak with a friend of mine, Sorrel King. Her daughter died of

mistakes here a few months ago and she is interested in improving safety."

I was not involved in Josie's care and had not even heard of Sorrel
or Josie, but was interested in talking with someone who understood
firsthand the importance of patient safety. Shortly after the talk,
David called Sorrel and told her that he knew a physician at Hopkins who was trying to make the hospital safer. She was encouraged
by this news and told David that she would like to arrange a meeting
with me, so he paged me with her number.

I called Sorrel and immediately sensed anger and sorrow in her
voice, but mostly anger. We spoke for about an hour. I explained
my ideas about the need to bring science to the delivery of care and
to improve patient safety so that another tragedy like Josie's didn't
happen again.

Sorrel invited me to come to her house to meet her husband,
Tony, and talk some more. A couple of days later, I found myself
pulling into the Kings' driveway. Their house sat on seven acres of
land that included what appeared to be a full-size lacrosse field.
Alongside of the house a trampoline sat idle in the grass; around it
was strewn an assortment of toys. Sorrel had other children, but this
empty play scene looked sadly abandoned. I was likely projecting my
own emotions, but I felt I could sense the tragedy here.

I rang the doorbell. Sorrel answered, took one look at me, and
said in a dismissive tone, "David didn't tell me you were so young. I'm
not talking to any more young doctors. I think you should leave."

I looked her in the eye and, smiling, replied, "I might appear
young, but we're probably about the same age." In a more serious
tone I added, "Sorrel, I can assure you I have a strong commitment
to improving patient safety at Johns Hopkins. I am determined to
make sure what happened to your daughter never happens again."

Tony came to the door and invited me in. I followed Sorrel and her husband through the kitchen, where her three other children were sitting at the table doing homework. Passing a stove covered with steaming pots, we entered the dimly lit living room and sat in front of a small, smoldering fire. Once again I felt a sensation of loss. This room, which should have represented the happy center of family life, had the lugubrious feel of a funeral parlor. Sorrel's anger was palpable. I was not sure if she saw me as a savior, or a villain from the evil empire that killed her daughter, or a little of both. To be honest, I'm not sure how I felt either. My affiliation with Hopkins and my role as a doctor brought with it a lot of guilt and, despite being from America's best hospital, shame. My institution, my colleagues, and even I were directly or indirectly responsible for Josie's death. Yet I was here on a mission to help make sure things like this never happened again. I was wearing two hats: one good, one shameful.

Feeling uneasy, I looked down at the end table, and I saw a picture of a little girl. I asked if it was Josie. When Sorrel replied in a shaky voice, "Yes," we both spontaneously started to cry. Looking at the photo of Josie, I felt as though I was looking at my own daughter, Emma, who was the same age and had almost the same smile, the same nose, the same eyes, and the same blonde hair. I imagined how I would feel if I had lost my daughter.

Sorrel's hard exterior softened. She and her husband told me about the series of events that led to their daughter's death and how they wanted to use some of their settlement from the hospital lawsuit to make a difference. I laid out my vision of how I planned to design, implement, and evaluate systems to improve culture and teamwork so we could learn from mistakes, not just recover from them. I told her how I wanted to train doctors and nurses in the science of patient safety. Tony and Sorrel liked the idea and were excited and encouraged to learn that someone was actively working to fix the broken system that they believed had killed their daughter. At that moment it was clear that they would do all they could to help me achieve this common goal.

I asked Sorrel to tell me about Josie. She said, "My daughter loved to bounce on the trampoline outside. She had just learned to say 'I love you.' She loved to wear dresses but always spilled food on them."

Sorrel's tone was still filled with anger, but I began to sense a few glimmers of hope. After talking for what must have been hours, she looked at Tony, then at me, and said, "Hopkins gave us money for what they did to Josie. We want to use that money to do something so this does not happen again. Hopkins had suggested we pay for a lecture on patient safety. We do not like that idea. We want to do much more. We want to do something that will save lives."

I suggested that the Kings use the money to support a safety team dedicated to the Johns Hopkins Children's Center where Josie had died. Sorrel could be part of the team, help design the interventions, and hold Hopkins accountable for improving care. I told them my wife, Dr. Marlene Miller, a pediatrician who did patient safety work, would be very happy to give her advice and guidance.

I explained that aside from her work as a Hopkins pediatrician, Marlene also obtained a degree in outcomes research and spent some time working with the Agency for Healthcare Research and Quality—the organization in the U.S. Department of Health and Human Services that supports quality and safety research. She was now helping the hospital's Department of Pediatrics with its safety efforts. She was and perhaps still is one of the few physicians with formal training in measuring and improving quality of care.

When I made this suggestion, energy filled Sorrel's defeated and drained body. She sat up and her voice became audibly louder and stronger. She asked if I thought this could really make care safer. It was clear she liked the idea.

"I have no doubt we can do a lot to make hospitals and health care safer," I told her. "It won't be easy; Hopkins is a great institution with a lot of brilliant minds. And most believe they are already providing excellent care, and often do. But the hospital can do so much more. And it will be hard to get people to see that, to get them to admit that they are still harming patients unnecessarily. It will make people uncomfortable and we may make some enemies along the way. It will require extra resources, yet I am certain we can make things better."

Sorrel held Tony's hand, and he looked at her as if it had been a while since they touched. She squeezed harder and asked me, "When can we start?"

I said, "Right away."

When I arrived home after leaving Sorrel and Tony, I sat with Marlene and told her of my visit, how Josie reminded me of Emma, and how we had to prevent what had happened to the King family from ever happening again.

I knew the best way to engage Hopkins in this work was to have Sorrel share her powerful story. Her tragedy made the statistics about the number of people who died from medical errors hauntingly real. The name Josie King could be the mnemonic touchstone that would inspire Hopkins to really focus on patient safety. I talked to my wife and the chairman of the Children's Center, George Dover, about having Sorrel form a special safety team for the Children's Center and they both thought it was a great idea. Sorrel and George both met with my wife and decided that Marlene would lead these efforts. We arranged to have Sorrel come and give a talk to doctors, nurses, and administrators at Hopkins. We wanted faculty and staff from the whole hospital to join. So we arranged to hold a special grand rounds and invited the whole hospital.

Of course this would never have happened if we didn't have approval from the Hopkins leadership. Hospitals typically don't invite the parent of a girl they killed to talk publicly. They consider the risk too high. I felt the risk was too high not to. Luckily, the administration had great vision in this regard. There was no question Josie's death had shocked Hopkins. The knee-jerk reaction for most medical institutions is to bury these types of errors, pay off whomever you have to pay off, and move on. However, our top leaders decided that instead of burying it, they wanted to talk about it and learn from it. Most importantly they didn't want anything like this to ever happen again.

"Josie's death had a huge impact on the institution and in some ways it allowed for a change of culture to occur," says the medical school's dean, Ed Miller. "There is a lot of arrogance in the institution; we believe we do no wrong, we are the world's greatest institution and so we don't make mistakes. I think we are changing that. It is painful when you screw up, but you have to say I really screwed up. Senior leadership has to say we are going to expose our mistakes."

We also had the full support of the Hopkins public relations team, the gatekeepers of Hopkins' public image, as well as support from the risk management department, the lawyers who work to prevent mistakes from harming patients and leading to lawsuits. They, like other Hopkins leaders, realized it was far better to face this problem and fix it than it was to sweep it under the rug.

When I asked Sorrel if she would come to Hopkins to tell her story, she was both excited and terrified. She had never given a talk in front of a large audience. She said she was not sure she could get through it and not really sure what she'd say. I was sympathetic. Nothing like this had ever happened, not at Hopkins, nor in the United States or even the world. Never had a hospital invited someone to come and talk about how their child was dead because of mistakes made by the hospital. Yet we believed that bringing Josie's story, and other medical errors, into the open would lead to healing and much-needed change at Hopkins.

Sorrel's initial fear turned into determination. She was soon drilling me about my research, asking how often people die from mistakes, what we knew about preventing errors, and what we were doing about it. I got her up-to-date on our work but cautioned her to focus mostly on speaking from her heart, not her mind. This audience did not need facts and figures. Hopkins is full of facts and figures. The staff needed to hear what it was like as a mother to suffer this kind of tragedy. I told Sorrel to let the memory of Josie guide her. The goals of her talk were to help everyone heal, to make this issue of patient safety real, and to generate passion and action to improve safety. In spite of my desire to downplay the event, this was a tall order for someone who had never given a public speech. Yet I saw power in Sorrel and power in her message; I knew she just needed to tap into her strength.

The morning of her talk she was fidgety and anxious. We grabbed a cup of coffee and entered Hurd Hall—the historic wood-paneled theater where so many world-renowned Johns Hopkins physicians and researchers had lectured over the years. Sorrel was wearing a blue business suit; her short, blonde hair was pulled back in a tight ponytail. She was a bit nervous but seemed well prepared. Mostly she seemed eager to deliver her message.

After I introduced her, Sorrel took the podium and the audience hushed. She began, "I am not a doctor or nurse. I am a mother who has seen the darkest side of medicine. My daughter Josie died here from preventable mistakes. I want to share my story with you in the hope that this does not happen again."

The power of her talk and the emotion in her voice grabbed everyone's attention. These administrators and doctors were used to tedious PowerPoint presentations laden with dry facts and figures; yet standing there before them onstage was this dynamic, energized, passionate, and tragic woman who was not methodically clicking through a series of dull slides nor speaking in abstractions. She was telling them a compelling, honest, personal story about what errors mean to patients and the families that love them. For most of her talk, Sorrel did not look up. She stood behind the podium and read from a script she held tightly in her hands as if it were an anchor against the rush of memory and emotion that swirled around her. Yet her message was clear, honest, heartfelt, and real. Many in the audience were tearful, including me.

I have heard Sorrel tell her story hundreds of times now, and I still tear up; perhaps it's because Josie reminds me of Emma, perhaps because of Sorrel's deep pain, or perhaps because I know we have a responsibility to prevent this from happening again.

At Hopkins and hospitals all over the world, we too often fall into the habit of looking at patient safety through the cold eyes of a statistician; lives become numbers and deaths becomes risk ratios. When you begin to understand how this work touches real people, when you can see the face behind the numbers, when you can feel the human suffering, it's powerful, and it changes everything. In the past my talks were laden with statistics, odds ratios, and confidence intervals. Today when I give a talk I come prepared with the facts, I know the statistics. But I have learned that it's real stories that move

people, not numbers or facts. There is no question you need to provide proof for your theories. But without the story, without emotion,
there is no context, it's just words.

Watching Sorrel tell her tragic story of error, death, and loss
was another defining moment for me personally, as well as for my
work in patient safety. Just as it was important to tell real stories,
I realized that we had to produce tangible results. What mattered
was saving lives, not just publishing papers. We needed to find a
way to engage doctors and nurses to make the changes necessary
to improve safety. If we don't engage and energize clinicians, if we
don't focus health care where it belongs, on the patient, then nothing will change. It is time for medicine to be held accountable. I was
not sure how we were going to get there, but I knew we had to find
a way to ensure that Josie and patients like her are less likely to die
today than last year, and that hospitals will be safer tomorrow than
they are today.

After the speech at Hopkins, Sorrel and Marlene went to work
trying to unravel what happened to Josie and how they could prevent
it from happening again. Sorrel joined me on many of my early safety
talks that I started giving around the country. We worked well as a
team: Sorrel touched hearts and I offered hope. This newfound relationship with Sorrel, and especially her story, gave me new direction
and drive in my work in patient safety. I was reminded, again, that
patients are suffering and dying and we have to do something to
change that.

One of the problems with health care that I knew was harming
patients was the lack of a good mechanism for getting proven treatments to the bedside where they can improve care. Determined to
study this problem, I went to work on a theory that is as basic as it
is complex. In its simplest form, it's essentially a checklist—a basic

to-do list like you might hang on your refrigerator. There's a wealth of medical knowledge out there that is simply not reaching patients; why not condense that knowledge into simple checklists that are easy for physicians to use?

This might sound obvious, too simple of an idea to solve the nation's health care crisis. Doctors are bound by the Hippocratic oath to try their very best not to harm patients. There is little to gain from cutting corners. So why do we need a checklist?

In the intensive care unit, where I worked as a new faculty member at that time, the average patient undergoes close to one hundred procedures a day (blood is drawn, heart rate is monitored, urine flow is measured), giving doctors two hundred to four hundred pieces of data (blood tests, X-rays, etc.) from which they must make scores of critical decisions. Life-or-death emergency procedures are daily occurrences, doctors are overworked, and ICUs are often crowded, hectic, and noisy. Furthermore, the way this work is organized, or in many cases not organized, often prevents patients from receiving the care they should; supplies are not stocked, labeling is ambiguous, communication is vague, absent, or confusing, and critical equipment is sometimes simply just not available, even at America's best hospitals.

Imagine a scenario in which a doctor can't find the bottle of chlorhexidine—an antiseptic solution she needs for a procedure. As she wanders around looking for it, one of the other patients in the ICU suffers a cardiac arrest and she offers assistance to that patient (emergencies like these happen quite often in the ICU). Once that patient is stable, she returns to her first patient but still does not have the antiseptic solution. At this point she's terribly behind schedule. She has many more patients to care for and has an important meeting with her department chief at the other end of the hospital.

She decides to forget about the chlorhexidine and just get the job done. From her perspective, this behavior is rational; she (like all of us) constantly makes trade-offs about risks and benefits. Time she spends looking for the antiseptic is time not spent with her patients. The care she can (or cannot) provide to other patients is visible and real while the infection that may develop from not using chlorhexidine is invisible and uncertain—most patients probably won't get infected, but some will. Yet this seemingly rational decision put this patient at risk.

Scenarios like this play out in hundreds of hospitals across the country every day. And although not using chlorhexidine when required will not result in infections in all patients, these infections can be very serious for the critically ill patients we treat in the ICU; they can even kill, especially bloodstream infections associated with the placing of a central line catheter.

Central line catheters, also called central lines, are used regularly in the ICU. They can, and often do, save a life. For example, these catheters make it possible to administer epinephrine directly to a patient's heart, a form of treatment used to stop cardiac arrest. They can also give physicians early warning that a patient is experiencing dangerously low blood volume in his heart, which could lead to shock, or they can tell us when a patient is going into heart failure, saving precious seconds and potentially avoiding death. Conversely, these catheters present a risk. It's estimated that the national mean rate of infections from central line catheters is four see p. 24 infections per thousand catheter days (a catheter day is one day that one patient has a catheter). That means each year roughly eighty thousand patients become infected as a result of placing central lines, and thirty thousand to sixty thousand die, at a cost of up to $3 billion nationally.

Yet although there have been an exhaustive number of studies that clearly outline proven techniques for preventing infections when inserting these catheters and the Centers for Disease Control and Prevention (CDC) produces guidelines summarizing this evidence, doctors don't use them. In fact, there is no standardized procedure for placing central lines that medical schools teach to students or that hospitals enforce in ICUs. Each doctor places central lines the way he or she happened to be taught, and if busy—which they always are—improvises.

Once we hired a nurse practitioner to work in the cardiac surgical ICU. As part of her orientation and training, the senior residents were supposed to teach her how to place central lines. This nurse practitioner came to me distraught and said, "Peter, can you help me? I am trying to learn how to place central lines. One resident showed me one way, but when I worked with a second resident, he said it was completely wrong and that I should only do it his way. Which one is correct?"

This lack of standardization is entirely unacceptable and dangerous to patients, yet it happens every day, across the country and around the world. It's obvious that everyone should receive the same evidence-based training, yet there is no system in place to guarantee all doctors will learn how to do it correctly. We need to find a way to make the latest medical research available and easily accessible to both the country doctor working in a small community hospital and the world-renowned surgeon working at a top medical institution like Johns Hopkins. Under the current model, students watch a procedure, they do it once, and then they are supposed to be able to teach it—often referred to as the "see one, do one, teach one" model. Instead of learning from the entire body of medicine, these students are only getting knowledge from one or perhaps two doctors; and there is no way of knowing if they are learning the correct procedure. In this way incorrect procedures might get passed down, unchecked, through generations of physicians, creating a chain of potential errors.

In modern medicine it's simply not acceptable to have a physician routinely doing it his or her "own way," blind to the possibility of newer, better methods. The approach may have worked a hundred years ago when medical research was in its infancy and many doctors worked alone with a simple black bag filled with a handful of therapies. In those days what a doctor "learned" through his own practice was often the best information he could draw from. Today, however, care is delivered by large teams of nurses, doctors, and technicians from a wide range of disciplines. Billions of dollars are spent annually developing new medicines and procedures. But care teams are poorly organized, and they often exercise more competition than cooperation. Compounding the problem is the fact that many new medical discoveries are simply not reaching doctors and patients who desperately need them.

For today's doctor to stay up-to-date with the latest treatments, he or she would have to study an impossible number of published scientific studies for the hundreds of diagnoses they may treat or procedures they may perform, leaving little time to actually practice medicine. Even if doctors read twenty-four hours per day, seven days per week, they could not consume the sheer volume of published literature available. However, if we could distill this research into its most effective components, combine it with what physicians and nurses learn on the job, and produce a simple, easy-to-follow protocol that contains the most essential information needed to protect

patients from harm—a checklist—we might have something doctors, nurses, and patients actually find useful. We might also make
hospitals safer.

The idea of a checklist really started to make sense to me when
I was preparing to attend a seminar on patient safety and medical
errors in Salzburg, Austria. Among the long list of experts on safety,
I saw that James Reason would also be attending the seminar. On
the flight over, I read Reason's book *Managing the Risks of Organizational Accidents*, which contained detailed information about aviation safety programs—specifically the use of checklists to improve
safety.

Though familiar with the idea of using checklists in aviation, I
had never really examined the theory. I was captivated. The parallels
between aviation and medicine were striking. Decision, control, and
inevitably the safety of passengers and patients were relegated to one
individual—in aviation, pilots; in medicine, doctors. Both professionals were expected to master complicated equipment and science
that was constantly evolving and changing. And in both arenas, errors could easily result in death.

But there were also significant differences between medicine
and aviation. In aviation the general acceptance that humans are
fallible was fundamental to the checklist's success. Once this truth
had been universally accepted, the industry was able to design systems that could prevent or catch inevitable errors before they caused
harm, or minimize the harm from errors that were not identified.

The health care community, however, has difficulty admitting
that well-meaning, highly trained, competent doctors predictably
and continuously make mistakes. So, when errors inevitably happen, the event and everyone involved are shrouded in guilt, shame,
denial, and secrecy. Also, medicine is infinitely more complex than

aviation. The amount of information that a doctor must retain to practice medicine is mind-boggling. To put this in perspective, what a pilot needs to know to fly a specific aircraft, say a Boeing 747, is the equivalent of what a doctor must remember to perform one single procedure. However, in a given week a physician will likely be called upon to perform hundreds of different procedures, whereas a pilot will most likely only need to know how to fly a couple of different aircraft. Similarly, every patient is different, and as such requires different treatment, knowledge, and skills, yet all 747s are pretty much identical. Also the number of new medical research studies far outweighs the number of new aviation studies published each year, which means more and more information keeps getting piled onto these overworked doctors. Finally, the aviation industry also keeps better records than we do in medicine, making it easier to monitor performance, standardize practice, and learn from mistakes. Keeping track of errors in aviation is much less complex than it is in medicine. In aviation all crashes are deemed preventable. Generally a healthy person boards a plane healthy. If passengers are killed, it is preventable. In hospitals people come to us already sick, many on the edge of death. If they don't survive, it is difficult to determine whether it was the result of an error or inevitability. Some patients are going to die, no matter how hard doctors and nurses try to save them. Separating preventable from inevitable harm requires science.

However, in spite of these challenges, I was intrigued by the similarities between aviation and medicine. It was clear we could learn a lot from the airline industry and I was convinced checklists in aviation were a good model for medicine. All that was required was some fine-tuning to accommodate the idiosyncrasies inherent to health care. To test my theory, we chose to use checklists to reduce the number of central line infections. These infections are common, costly, and often lethal. Most physicians believed deaths from infections were inevitable; they were the result of patients being sick or old or very young, or from having a complicated operation. Yet I knew that patients were not reliably receiving the interventions to prevent infections. And therefore, I believed they could be prevented. It wasn't practical to measure lives saved since patients in the ICU often die from a complex combination of factors and it is hard to definitively point to a central line infection as the exact cause of death. Furthermore, not all central line infections result in death. Only about one out of five patients with central line infections die. So it made much more sense to measure infection rates since there was no doubt that lowering these rates made patients safer, our ultimate goal.

When I began this work I was an attending intensivist in the surgical intensive care unit (SICU). (An intensivist is a primary care physician for very sick people, and "attending" meant that I was one of the senior-ranking physicians.) The SICU was a fifteen-bed unit staffed by critical care fellows, residents from the departments of surgery and anesthesiology, and nurses. Most of our patients were recovering from surgeries performed in the general operating rooms for vascular surgery, kidney and liver transplants, and trauma-related injuries. Like all ICUs, our patients were very sick and need the highest possible care and monitoring available. Our goal was to make them well enough so they could be transferred to a regular hospital bed and eventually sent home.

I chose the SICU for this study because I worked there—I knew the systems, I knew the procedures, and I knew the culture. More importantly, I had established strong relationships with this team, and I knew they were devoted clinicians that would do their best to support this effort.

Furthermore, the SICU was struggling with central line infections. If we were successful we would not only prove our system was effective, we would also save lives, and that was the ultimate goal. If we had tried to start this work somewhere else, it might not have even gotten off the ground.

# Chapter 2

See p. 17

In 2000, when I first began working in the SICU, the median rate of infections was 19 per 1,000 catheter days, giving us one of the worst records in the country.

Whenever we talked about improving this infection rate, the response from most of my colleagues was, "There is nothing we can do about it. Our patients are sick, we do big operations, and our patients are in the ICU for long periods of time." To be honest, a part of me believed that, too.

Physicians and nurses across the country conveniently place these infections and the consequential deaths into what I call the "inevitable bucket." Such deaths in a hospital are deemed unavoidable— chalked up to the cost of doing business. Sometimes this assumption is correct; large medical centers like Johns Hopkins tend to receive the sickest patients, some of whom might die in spite of receiving the best possible care. However, this is not true for all the patients who are dumped into this bucket. We really can't be sure how many of these infections are inevitable and how many are preventable.

What we did know was that a number of simple procedures had already been proven to prevent infections from central line catheters and in the SICU we were not using all of these consistently. In fact, at the time only around 30 percent of patients in America's hospitals, including Hopkins, were receiving the recommended measures to prevent central line infections. With such a low compliance rate, I was sure we could eliminate most of the infections if we followed these recommended practices. And if we could prevent these infections, many more patients would survive.

With this goal in mind, we worked closely with our hospital epidemiology and infection control colleagues and set out to create our first medical checklist. Infection control specialists study and track these infections, but do not place central lines. We recognized that in order to effectively reduce infections, these specialists would have to partner with the doctors whose job it was to place catheters.

Our plan was to include what we thought was a manageable number of key steps for doctors and nurses to follow to ensure patients did not get infections from catheters. We wanted to select steps that had the largest impact on reducing infections and the lowest risk to patients and costs. To this end, we sifted through reams of scientific evidence.

Much of this evidence is contained in the CDC's 120-page guidelines for preventing central line catheter infections—an enormous and comprehensive tome that offers an extensive and detailed outline of all the procedures that need to be followed to prevent catheter infections. This reference text is a scholarly summarization of the latest medical information for preventing this type of infection. It is thorough and unbiased and if followed, would most likely reduce central line infection rates.

However, it has a number of shortcomings. For one, while the format might be useful as a general reference, 120 pages of instructions listing scores of recommended procedures is not a practical reference guide for a busy clinician, especially since it does not prioritize what's most effective, most costly, or least risky. In a busy hospital it's not possible to sift through all the procedures listed in this guide, and it's certainly not possible or practical to attempt to perform all of them.

In addition, when evidence is incomplete (which is the norm rather than the exception), recommendations are often ambiguous. A common phrase that accompanies many of the recommended procedures in the guideline is, "Evidence is insufficient to vote either for or against." While this phrase might accurately summarize a lack of hard evidence regarding a procedure, it can be confusing and often not helpful to a physician. When facing a crisis we don't have time to decipher vague statements. Often a patient's life hangs in the balance. We have to make decisions, and we often have to make them fast. And even when we do have time, not making a decision is not an option.

Also, guidelines like this quickly become out-of-date. It requires an enormous amount of resources and money to produce them; they can take as much as a year to create and are updated (if at all) generally only every three to five years. Yet new studies are published daily, new information continues to accumulate, and these guidelines quickly become obsolete or inaccurate.

Another shortcoming of these guidelines is they lack "tacit knowledge." One of the greatest sources of knowledge in medicine comes from what physicians and nurses learn on the job. When questions arise about the care of a patient, doctors and nurses talking in the lounge or in conferences or at local meetings discuss and share how they treat various diseases and how patients respond to these treatments. This tacit knowledge develops and spreads into a "tribal knowledge" of techniques that work, and these techniques are soon practiced by a number of physicians and nurses. Much of this wisdom is not from the published literature, and some of it might not be very effective, but it is one of the ways physicians learn. This wisdom represents years of experience. If you pool all physicians, this adds up to thousands of years of collective knowledge. However, there is no existing system for capturing this knowledge and sharing it with the medical world, at least not yet. As a result, this important wealth of information is generally not included in guidelines.

It's obvious we needed a better system for translating scientific evidence into practice. These cumbersome guidelines must be combined with tacit knowledge and reduced to an unambiguous, behaviorally specific checklist that is high impact, low risk, cost effective, and, most importantly, *time efficient*. In our work, we sought to keep the checklist to seven items or less. The human brain has a hard time remembering more than seven items (for instance, any number longer than a phone number). And we cannot always count on physicians having immediate access to an electronic or paper copy of the checklist.

So our team sifted through the CDC guidelines, talked to nurses and doctors, observed how they placed central lines, and settled on five key steps:

- Wash your hands using soap or alcohol prior to placing the catheter.
- Wear sterile gloves, hat, mask, and gown and completely cover the patient with sterile drapes.
- Avoid placing the catheter in the groin if possible (these have a higher infection rate).
- Clean the insertion site on the patient's skin with chlorhexidine antiseptic solution.
- Remove catheters when they are no longer needed.

We distributed the checklists to doctors and then asked nurses to observe the rate at which doctors complied with the list. What we found was shocking. We had a dismal 38 percent compliance with the checklist—putting two out of three patients at greater risk of infection and death.

We knew the SICU would continue to have a lot of infections unless we somehow managed to persuade doctors to follow all the steps on the checklist all the time. I met with the doctors and nurses in the ICU and said, "Look, I know it is hard to say how many of our infections are preventable and how many are inevitable, but we know these five steps in the checklist will prevent a lot of infections. And we also know we're only using all of the steps 38 percent of the time. Could we make sure all our patients receive all of the checklist steps? Then we can see if it has any effect on the infection rates. It may or may not work, but my hunch is that we are going to see dramatic results."

As soon as I finished speaking, one of the doctors replied, "Peter, in a perfect world that would be fine, but it takes time to find all the things I need to perform those steps. And I don't have the time to run around the hospital looking for them."

I worked on the unit, so I knew that all of the doctors, including myself, were well intentioned: they wanted to provide the best care possible to patients. Yet they were incredibly busy, overworked, tired, and stressed and sometimes neglected to do all they were supposed to in order to protect patients against infections. This was not out of malice but rather for practical reasons; sometimes doctors thought it was not necessary, some did not know what they were supposed to do, sometimes it was difficult to use the checklist because the supplies were not available, and other times doctors simply forgot. A layperson would think that this couldn't happen, but when there's a lot going on, either because of an emergency or simply a high volume of work, and a doctor is being pulled six different ways, it's easy to skip a step. If he or she can't find a mask and gown, the doctor has to search for them or go without. Given the workload, time spent scrambling around looking for the needed equipment may injure other patients. Similarly, performing the procedure without the proper gear could also harm patients. The only acceptable solution was to ensure the supplies were available and that they were used.

I paused and thought about this. I worked in this unit and put central lines in all the time. Yet I couldn't remember not being able to locate the necessary supplies. So I ran a little test. The next time I had to place a central line, I paid close attention to the process. What I found was shocking. I had to go to eight different places to get all the items needed to comply with the checklist—caps we stored in one place, masks in another, gowns in yet another. To make things even worse, many items were altogether missing. I hadn't noticed it before because I had gotten used to running around; I did lines so often, the process had become automatic. I had gotten used to working in a dysfunctional system.

Next I observed my colleagues placing lines and learned they, too, had to travel all over the ICU to get what they needed. If they couldn't locate it easily, they generally paused a second and proceeded without the needed equipment. I stopped one of the doctors and asked why he was skipping a step. His response was, "I have a lot of patients to care for. If I spend too much time on this patient I won't have time for the others."

In his mind, he made a risk-benefit decision against complying with the checklist. He made a decision that the greater good was served by skipping a step. When doctors have to search for supplies, it adds more steps to the process. And with each added step, the risk of failure increases.

The solution was simple. We created a "central line cart" and stored all of the supplies needed to complete the checklist in one place. We asked doctors what they needed, decided what would be stored in the cart and on which shelves, and assigned someone the responsibility of keeping the cart stocked at all times.

We ran the test again and asked nurses to track performance. Compliance jumped from 38 percent to 70 percent. This was clearly an improvement, but it wasn't good enough. We needed compliance to be at 100 percent to see if the checklist was effective in lowering infection rates, and we weren't sure how to get there.

It was around this time that Sorrel King came to Hopkins to give a follow-up talk. It had been four years since Josie died. This time she was much more relaxed, she wore more casual clothes, she spoke freely from notes rather than reading from a script, and she challenged the audience to do more. The anger was still there but it was more controlled; she seemed better at using it to communicate and spur action. Sorrel and I had given a lot of talks together and she had also given a lot of speeches for the Josie King Foundation—a nonprofit she formed to help promote patient safety. (I served on its board.)

We met afterward and chatted as we often did when we met up on the road. But then suddenly, midsentence, she turned to me and asked me point-blank if I thought Hopkins was safer for patients. Excited about the work at Hopkins and eager to impress upon her that we were improving safety, I explained how we had put the checklist into play and standardized some of the procedures. I explained how we had some preliminary success at improving compliance. I tried to sound positive, but she didn't seem impressed.

She looked at me, her intense blue eyes piercing me like a scalpel, and said, "Peter, can you tell me Josie would be any safer at Hopkins now than she was four years ago? Look, I know you have all these hotshot docs here at Hopkins; I know you are all superbright, the top of your class. But you still make mistakes, and sometimes your egos lead you to make even more mistakes. What are you doing to fix those egos? In my definition of safety there is no room for egos. I don't care what you are saying. I want results. I want to see the evidence."

She had never been so direct or so abrupt. Perhaps being back at Hopkins, where it all started, where Josie died, was having an effect on her. Whatever it was, she was right on target and I knew it. In medicine, egos kill, and top hospitals, like Hopkins, certainly have their share of egomaniacs.

A couple of months before my meeting with Sorrel I was on call at home and got an urgent page at around ten p.m. from the surgical ICU telling me they had a very sick patient. I called the surgery resident and he gave me a quick history. The twenty-nine-year-old patient had been admitted the day before, in near-perfect health, to have a laparoscopic procedure to remove a kidney. However, shortly after the surgery it was discovered that the patient wasn't producing urine, a telltale sign of total kidney failure. The resident explained that the surgeon, convinced that his work had been flawless, gave the patient intravenous fluids in an attempt to kick-start her remaining kidney and get it working. It did not work; even after the patient had received twelve liters of IV fluids in ten hours (a tremendous amount) her kidneys were not producing urine. The surgeon ordered a CT scan and found some fluid in the pelvis (which could be common after surgery) but said the scan was otherwise normal. Bolstered by this report, the surgeon still believed the patient was fine, but just to play it safe he requested a bed in the intermediate care unit. Intermediate care units (IMCs) are way stations between ICUs and regular floor beds. IMCs have more nursing care than regular units but less than ICUs; they're for patients who are perhaps not sick enough for the ICU but nonetheless need more careful monitoring and special care than can be provided on a regular floor. As the intensive care physician on call, I assigned patients to IMC beds; however, the Department of Surgery was in charge of caring for the patients there. I asked the resident what he thought was wrong with the patient, he said, "I don't know but I think the patient will be fine; her surgeon just wants her to be closely monitored."

At around two a.m. I got a second page at my house from the surgical resident. I called him back and he requested that we admit this patient to the ICU immediately. The resident said the pH balance in the patient's blood was very acidic—a life-threatening condition; her belly was severely bloated (from all the fluid they were pumping into her that had nowhere to go); she was having difficulty breathing and needed to have a breathing tube placed; and her blood pressure was dropping rapidly. Bottom line, the patient was critically ill and needed care immediately or she might not make it. This once healthy woman who came to Hopkins for relatively routine surgery was now going to die, most likely from a medical error. I said to the resident that this patient needed to go to the operating room. She clearly had a problem related to her recent surgery. The resident told me the surgeon, who had gone home, maintained there had been no problem with the surgery and he would not take the patient to the operating room. I believed she needed to go to the OR and that, without surgery, she would die. I called the surgeon who had done the procedure, told him what I had learned about the patient from the resident, and advised that the patient needed to be taken to the operating room.

To my surprise, the surgeon's response was indignant. Clearly annoyed that I had called him, he said, "The CT scan was normal and I have full confidence in the surgery. There is no possible way I did anything wrong, and there is no reason for me to take her back into the operating room. We did the procedure laparoscopically using internal cameras and saw everything. It all went perfectly; there was no mistake."

My response was, "I understand the CT scan was normal but test results are not 100 percent dependable; we can sometimes have misleading CT scans."

Tests in medicine are generally good but they are not perfect. A small percentage of the time a CT scan is read as normal when the patient is sick and read as abnormal when the patient is fine. Doctors need to recognize this and when the evidence suggests that the test is wrong, they need to follow intuition and adjust care accordingly.

I said to the surgeon, "There was no medical condition that could make this happen, especially in this short a time. The only explanation for these symptoms, and how quickly she deteriorated, is a surgical complication. I know her CT scan was negative, yet these tests are not perfect. Everything else points to a surgical complication."

The surgeon literally yelled back at me over the phone, "There is no way this is a complication related to my surgery. I'm not taking her to the OR. The CT scan was normal and everything in the OR went perfectly."

I grew frustrated. I believed the surgeon was making a classic diagnostic error. But I also knew that if this turned into a battle of wills and egos, the surgeon (who was technically in charge of this patient) would harden up even more and refuse to compromise even an inch, and the patient would most likely die.

I rubbed the sleep out of my eyes, collected my emotions, and tried again, saying, "We are obviously seeing things differently here. Can you explain to me how you are weighing the risks and benefits of not going to the OR? I may be wrong, yet I see a healthy young woman who had surgery less than twenty-four hours ago who is dying because something bad seems to be going on in her abdomen. There is no medical condition that could cause this. I am asking you to go to the OR. If I am wrong, she has a scar. If you are wrong, she dies. What are you seeing that I am not?"

The surgeon amped up the volume in his voice and screamed back, "I am not going to the OR. I have to leave town. From now on, talk to the surgeon on call."

At that point, I knew our conversation was over. But he had given me an opportunity to save this patient. Up to this point I had to respect this surgeon's authority with regard to his patient; now that authority had shifted to the surgeon on call. Hopefully I would be able to get the surgeon on call to take this patient to the operating room. I knew I first needed to examine the patient myself to get accurate data and get a clearer picture, so I drove to the hospital. When I arrived at the ICU, the patient was dying, and I knew she was dying needlessly. When patients have severely distended abdomens, they are at risk for developing abdominal compartment syndrome, a condition in which the pressure in the abdomen increases and limits blood flow to the kidneys and intestines. It also compresses the diaphragm, often resulting in respiratory failure. Doctors diagnose this syndrome by measuring the pressure in the patient's bladder. I found the pressure in her bladder was very high and her remaining kidney and bowels were not getting enough blood flow; if these organs died, so would she. I was sure the compartment syndrome was being caused by some other problem and I suspected it was related to her surgery. But that didn't matter as much at this point. When a patient has abdominal compartment syndrome, you have to take her to the operating room; there is no other treatment. I contacted the surgeon on call and explained what had happened and told him the patient needed to go to the operating room for surgery or she would die. This surgeon, thankfully, did not argue with me and took the patient to the operating room. As soon as the patient was opened we discovered that my suspicions were correct. During the previous surgery the trocar, a harpoonlike rod used during laparoscopic surgery, had accidentally punctured her intestine and her pancreas. Accidents like this happen; surgery is not a perfect science. However, if this had been discovered quickly the patient might have suffered less harm. But thanks to arrogance and abstinence, this life-threatening injury had been undiscovered for eighteen hours, resulting in the patient losing her remaining healthy kidney. The patient, who should have been released after three days, spent six months in the hospital until she was finally discharged, only to spend another year in rehab. This healthy woman who had come into Hopkins at 110 pounds now weighed 80 pounds, had had a tracheotomy, could barely speak or walk, and was on dialysis and needed a kidney transplant, all needlessly.

Hopkins is one of the best medical centers; we have some of the best surgeons in the world. Errors like this are not generally made from a lack of technical expertise but rather from bad teamwork and a toxic hospital culture, something that is endemic to the entire health care system.

As this terrible experience flashed across my memory, I had no choice but to look Sorrel square into her blue eyes and say, "You're right, arrogance kills and we need to weed it out."

She answered, "Enough already, Peter. We already know this is a problem. How do you know you're making it better? I want to know, if Josie were admitted today, would she be less likely to die? I want to know health care is safer. It damn well better be."

My hands were sweating; my stomach churned. I knew I did not have the results to tell Sorrel what she wanted to hear. We only had 70 percent compliance for our checklist, and that was only for one procedure out of hundreds we perform daily in the SICU, let alone the rest of the hospital. I also knew we had a culture in health care that was, in many ways, toxic. Doctors often think they are infallible, communication between doctors and nurses is poor, and accountability is virtually nonexistent. We have few valid measures of patient safety and these often are not made available to the public. I looked at Sorrel, disillusioned despite all my hard work, and said, "I don't have an answer, but I promise you I will."

As the words left my mouth, I knew they were wholly inadequate. I knew she deserved an answer; I knew my family deserved an answer; I knew every patient who walks into a hospital or visits his or her doctor deserves an answer. Yet neither I, Johns Hopkins, nor the U.S. health system had a clue whether safety was improving.

Sorrel had exposed one of the key problems with health care and my current research. Patient safety efforts wouldn't make a dent unless doctors changed the way they practiced medicine. We needed a collaborative culture so that we could redesign systems. Without that, our checklist would be just another good-intentioned New Year's resolution that failed. Except this was not a diet or exercise program; it was patients' lives.

I reflected on the issue for a long time before it suddenly hit me: the checklist wasn't working because I put doctors in charge of themselves. Given doctors' overloaded schedules, the complexity of modern health care, and especially their inflated egos and overconfidence, it wasn't realistic to expect them to obey a checklist that was being imposed on them. Doctors needed someone to remind them to follow the steps and hold them accountable. Doctors had to acknowledge they were fallible and work with the team to ensure patients did not needlessly suffer.

We needed an independent observer who could reliably ensure that none of the steps were overlooked. If one or two were skipped, the observer would be there to remind the doctor about the checklist and insist that the steps be completed. The observer would need to be empowered and have support. Given that a patient's life is at stake, this approach makes sense—it actually seems more like a moral issue than a political or scientific one. But sadly, and surprisingly, doctors are often not receptive to taking instruction from anyone, not even another physician, let alone a nurse. I was starting to get close to the root of the problem that has been keeping hospitals in the dark ages and derailing our attempts to improve safety. Hospitals suffer from an antiquated and often toxic culture that creates and supports broken systems that, in turn, harm patients. Without a change in culture we would not be able to improve those systems and patients would continue to be in danger.

In 1991, when I was a medical student, I was asked to work in a mission hospital in Ogbomosho, Nigeria. Sorely underfunded, it consisted of a collection of low, cinder-block buildings surrounded by a tall security wall. The patient wards were like barracks—row after row of dusty mattresses on metal-framed beds spaced two feet apart, with no private rooms and no curtains. The electricity went out every day for hours, and the hospital didn't have enough fuel to keep its emergency generators running. There was no air-conditioning, only ceiling fans that stopped working when the power went out. The heat was often oppressive and only exaggerated the ever-present odor of sweat, blood, urine, and infection.

The hospital had a large walk-in clinic. Most of the patients had broken bones from motor vehicle accidents that needed to be set, dysentery from bad water, or abscesses that needed to be cut and drained. The other common injury was burns, mostly from the open fires used to cook food and boil water, or from lighted cans of oil the villagers would carry on their heads in order to see at night since electricity was scarce.

I started my day making rounds in the barracks before going to the clinic. In one of the beds lay a young boy whose eyes still haunt me today. He had third-degree burns on his legs that went down to ligaments and bones; the skin was entirely missing and the bones and ligaments were infected. He smelled of rotting burned flesh. He was awake, and I was sure he was in pain but he did not show it; like many people who are chronically exposed to suffering, he was resilient and stoic. His deep brown eyes looked frightfully at me. His father, a proud man, barely thirty but with rotting teeth and foul breath, stood next to him. His face was blank. He did not hold his child's hand to provide comfort, nor did he show much compassion or emotion.

The boy's only chance for survival was amputation. His legs were too burned to heal and, without an amputation, the infection in his legs would spread to his blood and kill him. But in Ogbomosho (and much of the developing world), there's little or no work even for healthy people, and amputees often end up as beggars, something the child's father would not permit. I tried to talk to him. I explained that without amputation his child would not survive, but it was no use. He looked at me steely-eyed and simply said, "No operation." The father would rather watch his son die than suffer the shame of having his son become a beggar.

Eventually the inevitable happened. The boy's infection spread to his blood and slowly sucked the life out of him. On his last night, I stayed up with the unlucky child. I held his hand through the night and watched his eyes change from fearful to peaceful, as death slowly came and carried him away. Initially he clutched my hand as if he were trying to pull my life energy into his, then his grip slowly lessened. This was the second time I had held a death vigil (the first with my father) and in both cases, the deaths need not have happened.

Watching that child die needlessly, along with hundreds of other tragedies I witnessed while working in that clinic, taught me that success, as a doctor, was not singularly dependent on hard work or even my individual skill as a doctor. Culture, and the systems it influences and creates, can have an even larger influence on patient outcomes. In the United States this child would have lived and probably had a fruitful life, but in Ogbomosho, because of the poverty and the attitudes of his father and the local society, he did not receive the necessary and available treatment. Culture got in the way.

To improve health care, we need to examine how culture affects the systems and structures within which we do our work. Culture influences how we deliver care, how we interrelate with our colleagues, and how we treat our patients. Similarly, the systems in which we work and live, in turn, affect culture—they are interconnected. Whether in a clinic in Africa or in the halls of an American hospital, culture and systems must be reevaluated in order for patient safety to be achieved.

In an article published by the journal *Annals of Internal Medicine*, I described an incident in which a junior resident once pulled a dialysis catheter out of a patient's neck while the patient was in a sitting position. The patient then suffered an air embolism, where air enters and stops the heart, and needed to be resuscitated. Upon reviewing the case, the first reaction of the chief resident and the attending physician was to scold the junior resident—"Why did you remove the catheter when the patient was sitting? You know we are not supposed to do that!" Their anemic remedy was to put an incident report in his file that admonished him to be more careful and not do it again. This is a typical but wholly ineffective approach to solving problems like these.

Let's look more closely at this error. The resident was obviously not properly trained. The other doctors present at the time didn't ask the junior resident if he knew what he was doing, which effectively enabled him to make the error. Why wasn't there a checklist for how to do this procedure properly? Why wasn't the doctor properly supervised or previously evaluated and deemed competent? Similarly, the nurse who was standing by the junior resident's side watched while he made the error, but said nothing. When the nurse was asked why she didn't speak up, she said the last time she said anything, she got her "head bitten off" by the doctors. She didn't want to be in that position again, so she stayed silent, even though it endangered the patient's life.

The truth is that it wasn't entirely the junior resident's fault. He was a victim of an outdated hospital culture in serious need of reform. He trained under the antiquated model—see one, do one, teach one—used by all health care institutions. As a result, he probably only saw it performed once and was not sure exactly how it was done. The culture of perfection among physicians often discourages young doctors from asking questions because it might make them look stupid or mediocre to their superiors and they are deathly afraid of being humiliated—a daily occurrence. So this resident decided to avoid that humiliation and took a chance that he would get it right. He was wrong and he almost killed his patient.

Junior doctors need training. And that training will include a learning curve, yet this process should not put patients in harm's way. A system that exposes a patient to potential harm as part of a doctor's education is unacceptable. The whole purpose of residency is to practice in front of a professional so the more experienced physician can teach you and catch errors before they harm patients. However, if the toxic culture of a hospital setting makes it so a resident is afraid to ask questions of a senior doctor, or a nurse does not speak up when he or she sees someone putting a patient at risk, this educational model fails and, worse yet, places patients at great risk.

This type of scenario plays out all the time, in every hospital multiple times a day. When I had finished my residency and was doing my fellowship to become an intensivist, I decided to take a breathing tube out of a patient. I thought the patient would be fine without it, but I was wrong: the patient needed the tube. By the time we got the tube back in, the patient had suffered temporary brain damage. I later learned that the patient's nurse predicted that this might happen, but she did not speak up. And I did not ask her because I wanted to appear as if I knew what I was doing.

I will never forget watching the family react to the news—they were clearly devastated. Luckily the patient recovered, but he might not have. In any case I learned that it was not acceptable to routinely put patients at risk like this, and it was equally unacceptable to put family members through this kind of pain and agony.

Today, even though I am a senior physician, I routinely ask all members of the team their perceptions whenever making important decisions for a patient. In this way I try to tap the wisdom of the team. I know that I will make a wiser decision with broad input. This input does not compromise my authority; it enhances it. It doesn't matter how much training or skill I have, I can still make a mistake, so why take the risk?

What's really at play is not only a flawed system, but the age-old, unhealthy culture that created and perpetuates that broken system. This toxic culture is at the core of most hospital errors. Medicine, historically, has inhabited a rarified, almost sacred world where doctors assume godlike status. It's not surprising since physicians literally hold a patient's life in their hands. Yet, even though the stakes are clearly higher than in other professions, it is still a job performed by humans who inevitably will make mistakes. Physicians, patients, and nurses regularly make this mistake of assuming doctors have some kind of higher power. This false belief often discourages patients or clinicians from questioning doctors. In the same fashion, it can discourage physicians from questioning ourselves and asking for help—we are not supposed to need it. For years medicine has operated like a private club of self-styled deities where the entrance requirement is an M.D. The better the medical school or residency training program, the more prestigious the club, the more powerful the god. Considering the sacrifices doctors have to make to obtain a license to practice, it is easy to understand how this false kingdom was created. Similarly, it is understandable that physicians would be reluctant to let outsiders into the club, or listen to the advice of a nurse or a family member when it comes to patient care.

There is little question that someone needs to be in charge and claim responsibility for a patient's care, as well as make the final call. And since doctors have the most training, they are best suited for this role. Nobody is disputing that. However, it isn't wise to ignore the advice of nurses, family members, or patients, each of whom possesses valuable information that could help doctors better understand their patients and make better decisions.

Doctors need to recognize that formal education is important but it is not the only source of knowledge. Time spent suffering from a disease or time spent tending to or living with a patient suffering from a disease is also a valuable source of knowledge. Even though it may seem counterintuitive, sometimes patients and their families trump nurses and nurse trump doctors. Indeed, often the physicians themselves hold the lowest position on the experiential knowledge totem pole.

During our work on bloodstream infection in the SICU, I read James Surowiecki's book *The Wisdom of Crowds*. Surowiecki argues, rather convincingly, that an independent and diverse group can make better decisions than a highly trained and educated individual. Yet in medicine, doctors are taught to ignore the crowd and trust their own training and education. If Josie's doctors had embraced the "wisdom" of the crowd associated with Josie's care they might have made a better decision about Josie's treatment. Josie's mother's suspicions that her daughter was dehydrated proved accurate, but the surgeons, despite all of their training, apparently missed this and Sorrel's concerns were not addressed. Even more remarkable and disturbing, the surgeons also appeared to have ignored the pain physician, who was a highly trained and brilliant pediatrician and anesthesiologist. They also apparently did not heed advice from the nurses, who had considerable training and experience and arguably had the most accurate and up-to-date sense of Josie's condition since they had spent the most time with the patient. If these physicians had adjusted their care based on the full range of knowledge provided by every member of this extended team, Josie might have lived. However, a doctor is trained to trust his or her judgment first and foremost and discount everyone else's opinion in varying degrees, from fellow physicians all the way down to a child's own mother.

Each of the members of a patient's team, including a parent if the patient is a child, sees problems through a different set of lenses that is shaped by personal experiences and training. Each of those lenses provides valuable information, information that helps us make wise decisions. Nurses see things differently than doctors, junior doctors see things differently than senior doctors; patients see things differently than clinicians; and family members have their own lenses. No lens is more accurate than the other; they are just different. Each has a partially incomplete view of a complex puzzle. The fewer the lenses the more distorted the view, the worse the decision, and the greater the risk for preventable harm. A team approach does not detract from a physician's talent, authority, or power; it only enhances them by ensuring that he or she makes the best possible decisions. Ultimately, the lead physician should and will make the final decision about what therapies to offer and what tests to obtain. However, doctors who choose to make these decisions in a vacuum are exceedingly dangerous.

The point here is not to place blame on the doctors; that's too easy and also inaccurate. They are a product of the system that trains them, and as such, Josie's surgeons were simply following this training. Current medical training focuses on technical prowess rather than intrapersonal and interpersonal skills. Medical training, especially surgical training, is defined by years and years of competitive isolation. We produce autonomous physicians rather than team-oriented professionals. In order to get into the best schools, future doctors often forgo socializing and hit the books hard, often as early as high school. Once in medical school these doctors-in-training are in direct competition with their fellow students as they vie for the top positions; the same is true in residency. When physicians finally complete their training it's not always easy for them to turn this pattern around and start working with a team. This climate of competition only increases throughout their careers as doctors vie for better positions and more prestige. And it will remain unchanged until doctors are given instruction or support on how to learn these new skills.

There is no question in my mind that the doctors in charge of Josie King's case were good at their work. I am convinced they tried to give Josie the very best of care. It wasn't entirely their fault that things went wrong. The culture of medicine and the faulty systems that culture creates played a large part in this error. In many ways they were merely a product of that culture—and most likely blind to it. It is hard to see culture when you are in it.

In our patient safety studies that appeared in the *Annals of Surgery* and the *Journal of the American College of Surgeons*, my colleagues and I distributed a survey that gauged teamwork and communication in the operating room. Results revealed that almost all the doctors believe teamwork in the operating room is good and most think it is great, while more than half of the nurses think it is lousy. I was astonished. How can this be? These doctors and nurses work next to each other, in the same operating room, doing the same operations, yet their attitudes and perceptions are vastly different. We soon learned that similar discrepancies exist in every corner of the hospital and in every one of the hundreds of hospitals in which we measured culture.

When I graduated from medical school I believed that the definition of good teamwork is when a doctor gives a nurse an order, the nurse does it. Despite playing team sports throughout high school and college, I somehow forgot what I learned about collaboration. Medical school produced a view of teamwork that was more of a dictatorship than a dialogue.

One day on rounds a nurse had something to tell me, but I was busy. Obviously I didn't think it was that important. Luckily the nurse stopped me and said, "The patient's blood gas has severe metabolic acidosis." I looked into the nurse's eyes and realized that my naive attitude about nurses could have threatened this patient's life. She was telling me that some part of the patient's body was not getting blood flow. I immediately tended to the patient and we discovered that a section of his bowel was dying. If I had not acted quickly, this patient's condition would have deteriorated rapidly. He would have likely died. The nurse's advice did not take away my authority— quite the opposite. What it did was save me from making a costly and potentially deadly error. Needless to say, today I define good teamwork as doctors and nurses having clearly defined roles and responsibilities yet working interdependently, exchanging information and backing each other up in order to maximize the safety of the patient. Yet few medical and nursing schools train students in how to work effectively in teams, despite a wealth of evidence that has shown this is key to improving safety and quality of care. When I was in medical school I spent hundreds of hours looking into a microscope—a skill I never needed to know or ever use. Yet I didn't have a single class that taught me communication and teamwork skills—something I need every day I walk into the hospital.

Toxic hospital culture, and the training and systems that create it, not only negates effective teamwork, it also perpetuates a false and dangerous myth that doctors can't make mistakes. Though errors are inevitable, though fallibility is part of the human condition, young doctors are told they must perform flawlessly. A pulmonary catheter goes deep into the heart. If it goes too far, it could rupture the large blood vessels that lead to the heart. Physicians are supposed to know that this danger increases significantly when these catheters are inserted sixty centimeters beyond an entry point in a vein in the neck. Yet this potentially life-threatening error happens regularly. So why don't medical experts place a simple movable hub on the catheter—at sixty centimeters—that forces doctors to stop and think before inserting too far? The technical solution is relatively easy; but that change requires that doctors admit they will make mistakes. The culture says, *doctors know not to put it in too far, so they won't*. So the hub has never been developed.

Similarly, an estimated 750,000 people each year suffer a cardiac arrest in the hospital. Cardiac arrest is almost always treated with a defibrillator. Yet roughly 30 percent of the time, physicians operate these machines incorrectly. So why not redesign them so they are easier to use, or print clear instructions on the machine? Because no doctor wants to admit that he or she doesn't know how to use it correctly. No one wants to admit doctors are human, they are flawed, and they can make mistakes.

When I removed that breathing tube, the word "mistake" was never spoken. I had to suffer my shame alone, which is probably why I still carry the story around with me. That's just how we were trained to behave. Doctors, especially doctors at top medical institutions like Johns Hopkins, are not allowed to make mistakes. And we are taught not to talk about mistakes, as if denial somehow absolves their impact. I wasn't even able to apologize to the patient's wife, who had tears in her eyes. Yet, I wanted to.

Doctors carry mistakes like these around with them for years. In my talks on patient safety I started to pull back this curtain and dispel this erroneous myth. I conveyed the message that it's culture and systems, not bad doctors, that make these mistakes and that it's okay not to be perfect. Standing in front of my peers I admitted openly that I had made, and still make, errors. That admission seemed to open up the door and encourage my fellow doctors to speak about their mistakes—perhaps for the first time in their careers. It was like an emotional dam broke somewhere in health care.

Doctors shared stories of errors that harmed patients—errors they will never forget. Some of these stories were twenty years old. Many physicians got tearful as they talked, clear proof that the guilt and shame were still potent, potent because they were never addressed, because these people were led to believe they were somehow supposed to be perfect.

I knew that without changing these unhealthy patterns and backward systems, without a change of culture, our checklist would fail. But it wasn't going to be easy. These cultural dynamics have been a part of medicine for longer than anyone can remember, and they are especially prominent in older, prestigious medical centers like Johns Hopkins.

However, in the SICU where we were doing research, we had some leverage to change this culture. These were my colleagues, the people I worked with every day. We were addressing a committed team of physicians and nurses who were willing to try new approaches. Also, Josie King's death had gained me the support of the hospital administration—the need for patient safety initiatives at Hopkins had become paramount. That meant that not only the nurses, but also my fellow doctors in the ICU would be more encouraged to try a new approach, knowing the top executives were behind it. Support also meant that if we needed help from the Hopkins administration all we had to do was ask; if they agreed with our goals, they would make an effort to back us up with whatever political or economic resources were necessary.

We knew the only effective way to ensure that physicians followed the checklist was to have independent monitors with the authority to force doctors to comply. To accomplish this we were

SAFE PATIENTS, SMART HOSPITALS 49

going to have to shake up the culture; and for that we were going to take significant heat. We couldn't ask doctors to monitor doctors; we didn't have the staff for that. That left us only one choice: We would have to ask nurses to monitor doctors and make sure the checklist was followed religiously.

This was unprecedented. Never before had nurses been given this type of authority. Not only could a nurse correct a doctor if he made a mistake, but the nurse could also demand that the doctor immediately fix the error. When I presented this to the staff, the reactions from both doctors and nurses were brutal. It was like World War III.

Nurses rolled their eyes and said, "It is not my job to police doctors and even if I did, I would get my head torn off."

On the other side, doctors said, "I am not going to have a nurse question me in public; I will look like I don't know what I'm doing."

My response was, "Welcome to the human race. You don't know everything and you are not expected to."

What was striking was that nobody debated the evidence, nobody challenged the items on the checklist, and nobody questioned whether we should do them. But everyone objected to the change in culture. The doctors saw it as a loss—a loss of power and respect, a loss of all they had worked so hard in medical school and residency to achieve. The nurses also didn't trust this change. They felt it would open them up to abuse and criticism.

My job was to convince the doctors that by asking them to listen to the other members of the care team, I wasn't taking away authority, I was helping them to make better-informed decisions and therefore deliver a higher standard of care. I also had to convince the nurses that they played an important role in making sure patients received the best care possible and that I would guarantee they would be supported in exercising that role freely and with confidence.

I asked the nurses, "Is it tenable that we regularly put patients in harm's way?" Many shook their heads. "Then how can you sit and watch a doctor not follow the correct procedures, risking the patient's life in the process?"

Next, I turned to the doctors and said, "Let me make this really, really clear. Nurses will question you. If you make a mistake, you will go back and fix the problem the nurse identified. However awkward we might feel letting a nurse correct or question us, however fearful a nurse might be that a doctor will react badly to her advice, we have to keep remembering that it is *patient care* that is the goal here, not stroking egos or reinforcing an antiquated hierarchy. The patient is our 'North Star,' and every action we take ultimately must be guided by delivering the very best care to our patients. That's our bottom line. I do not expect you to be perfect; none of us ever will be. However, I do expect you to help create a system to ensure that patients always receive recommended therapies, that patients are not needlessly harmed. While individuals, even brilliant Johns Hopkins physicians, will always make mistakes, teams can perform much better."

To give my reforms some teeth, I told nurses to page me directly if a resident physician gave them any resistance. In addition, each of our top executives gave the ICU teams the same message: "Page me or call my cell phone if the doctors don't comply with the checklist."

The results were staggering. A year later, infection rates in the SICU had dropped nearly to zero. We saved an estimated eight lives and $2 million. In addition, neither I nor any of Hopkins' top administrators got a single page complaining that a doctor was not complying or behaving poorly.

The success of this program inspired everyone on the team. We had a poster on the wall tracking infection rates. The poster listed the quarterly rates of infections, as well as every week we went without an infection. As the rates dropped, the number of weeks got longer and the team got stronger and more eager to work hard at keeping them down. We knew we were onto something. Our only question now was, could we do it again? Was this just beginner's luck, an anomaly, or could we package this process and apply it successfully to other broken systems that were harming patients?

With this goal in mind, we took what we learned fighting central line infections and we created our first model for patient safety—a model that we hoped could theoretically reduce patient harm from other procedures. We knew our success would depend on three key elements: Developing an unambiguous checklist that encapsulated as much knowledge or evidence as we could gather on a particular procedure; changing the culture and associated broken systems to remove any barriers to implementing that checklist; and measuring results so we could gauge the checklist's efficacy and provide feedback to make whatever changes necessary to improve it.

The primary goal of our new model was to deliver the latest treatments to the bedside where they belong, so we decided to call it "translating research into practice," or TRIP. And though culture *TRIP* change and measurement were the essential elements that fueled TRIPs success, the vehicle for delivery was clearly the checklist.

# Chapter 3

We use checklists to standardize and ensure quality, consistency, and safety every day of our lives. Even something as ubiquitous as our morning cup of coffee comes with its own checklist.

- Choose the best water—coffee is 98 percent water, so the quality of the coffee is dependent on the quality of the water used.
- Match grind and coffee maker—each coffee-making process requires a specific grind, coarse for a French press, fine for espresso.
- Keep the coffee fresh—air, moisture, and sunlight harm coffee, so keep it properly stored.
- Use the correct proportions—it's best to use 2 tablespoons of coffee for every 6 ounces of water.

As simple as this sounds, coffee is complex—nowhere near as complex as the human body, but nonetheless complex. One could easily write a three-hundred-page book on how to best transform this scrubby little plant into a delicious, warm, eye-opening beverage. Roast, altitude, soil, sunlight, rainfall, and a slew of other factors all likely have some affect on the flavor. However, according to most coffee aficionados, when I wake up and prepare my morning fix, all I have to really concern myself with is four key elements—a checklist, if you will.

Successful companies have been using checklists for years to ensure quality. Important processes are trimmed down to manageable essential steps, standardized, and consistently performed. Yet this kind of standardization is sorely lacking in health care. Look at something as obvious as hand washing. Of all the ways in which hospitals could try to fight infections, hand washing is arguably the most effective. Yet doctors do not wash their hands consistently when visiting a patient and there is no standardized procedure in place to ensure they do. They know they are supposed to, but on average they do it 30 percent of the time. Perhaps more alarming, most hospitals do not monitor rates of hand washing and there's no accountability for this performance. And while people don't usually die from bad coffee, many patients have likely died from bacteria on a physician's hands.

Why isn't hand washing standardized in hospitals—along with thousands of other procedures that are known to save lives? It would be easy to blame doctors, but the bulk of the problem does not lie there. Most physicians care deeply about their work and want nothing but the safest care for their patients. It's the culture of medicine and the systems within which doctors practice that are at fault. Physicians, including myself, are trained to believe that we don't need standardization because we don't make mistakes; we are told that our brains have endless storage capacity and that we have perfect recall of all the thousands of hours' worth of information we've learned from medical school and years of practice. Yet we do not. The fact is, just like all other humans, we forget. We are fallible. We do not see systems and we are not trained to improve them.

Furthermore, doctors are also trained to believe that we don't always have to follow the rules or ask for anyone's help. We are the smartest people in the world and can figure out any problem on our own. When I was in medical school, I remember specifically being told, "Guidelines are for simple physicians, not Hopkins physicians. At Hopkins we know the evidence; we are expert clinicians; we know the nuances of our patients so we do not need guidelines." I have since realized how dangerous it is to use that statement to train physicians.

It's true every patient is unique and clear guidelines for some procedures or conditions are often absent or incomplete, making it necessary for doctors to rely on professional judgment to make personal, often independent, decisions about care. When evidence is immature or lacking, our intuition or reasoning is often the best evidence we have. However, we also need to recognize that standardization offers tremendous benefits, especially when evidence is robust. As medical science matures, we must progress from providing care primarily based on intuition, to a place where this independent approach is properly balanced with care based on collective wisdom and proven scientific evidence.

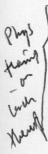

Yet as science continues to propel us into the future at an alarming rate, the culture of medicine dwells solemnly in the past. We do not train clinicians about the value of standardization, we do not train physicians to share knowledge or to improve bad systems that harm patients, we do not train physicians to work as a team organized around the patient, and for the most part we do not hold them accountable for their performance or patient outcomes.

Part of this lack of standardization is necessary; we want physicians to be innovative, to be always coming up with new treatments and therapies. Without this freedom to operate outside of convention, medicine would not advance, nor would many of its greatest discoveries even exist. Innovative medical procedures and an occasional breaking of the rules (such as letting a brilliant lab technician operate on humans) helped Johns Hopkins surgeon Alfred Blalock, cardiologist Helen Taussig, and laboratory technician Vivien Thomas develop the first "blue baby" surgery, which corrected a heart defect that was killing infants. Without similar innovation we could never have developed bypass surgery, transplant surgery, chemotherapy, angioplasty, imaging, many antibiotics—or any of the thousands of other medicines and medical procedures that keep people alive today.

However, these great discoveries are only effective if they reach patients, and there is no real system in place to ensure that an effective procedure developed in a lab will reach a small regional hospital. Is it acceptable that a patient dies needlessly simply because a doctor does not know the latest treatment for his condition? Every day, in every hospital in the world, good, even great doctors misdiagnose and mistreat patients because knowledge is not effectively shared between hospitals and physicians. In the United States patients are receiving barely 50 percent of recommended therapies. To remedy this imbalance, we need to standardize those treatments, provide easy access to the scientific evidence supporting them, and redesign our systems so we can incorporate them into our daily practice. Yet this is not happening, in part because health care suffers from a poor "knowledge market."

What is a knowledge market? The recent mortgage crisis that shook the entire world economy is a clear example of a poor knowledge market. In that case the risks of the large or unsecured mortgages were known by lenders, but not by the investment companies that were making bets on them. Greed compelled lenders to downplay those risks, and lax regulations made the risks invisible. All of this was compounded by well-intended federal policies that encouraged home ownership. In the end, valuable information was not shared with all participants and the whole thing fell apart.

Some may argue that this is the cost of doing business, buyer beware. But there are some goods, like mortgages, which are so important that society needs to take steps to ensure that all players are well informed. I certainly understand competition among mortgage companies, but they should be competing with all the cards on the table, not on hidden truths, misinformation, or downright lies. Medicine is equally, if not more, important to the health and success of society. To reduce preventable illness, death, and the rising cost of care, we need to create a better health care knowledge market. We need to make all existing knowledge transparently available.

We also need to increase the efficiency with which we gather and share knowledge. In health care we depend mostly on formal clinical studies. Yet less than 0.1 percent of patients are enrolled in these studies. For the other 99.9 percent of patients, we learn little or nothing. We need to collect and distribute what we can learn from all patients in real time, at the bedside. Yet we do not routinely monitor what we do or the results we achieve. So we cannot decipher what works or does not work or what might be harmful to patients.

There is no other industry where this would be tolerated. When medical knowledge is not shared, patients pay a terrifying price. The failure of medicine's knowledge market, the failure to deliver to all patients the accurate diagnosis and the treatments known to prevent death and disability, could very well be the leading cause of death in the United States.

TRIP brings teams together to study and share the abundant wealth and breadth of knowledge from both scientific research and the tacit knowledge that team members have learned on the job. That knowledge is distilled into a simple checklist that provides the latest up-to-date and most effective treatments and procedures.

However, checklists are useless if people don't use them, and people won't use them unless they own them. So instead of imposing a generic set of rules using the top-down management model that we already know doesn't work, we thought it better if we supply the evidence, give an example of a checklist, and have teams tailor their own checklists based on what's needed and what works for them, given the cultural dynamics and unique nature of each unit. The why, what, and how behind the checklist is shared and literally developed by the team through group discussions and the telling of real stories involving patient harm. Once teams have clarified the checklist, they need to systematically identify and mitigate barriers that prevent patients from receiving the interventions on the checklist. Next, teams need to monitor performance to see whether the checklist is used and/or whether patient outcomes improve. Finally, teams need to reorganize their work to ensure that patients always receive the items on the checklist.

Ownership is easily the most important aspect of TRIP. Doctors and nurses are busy people who are constantly given new procedures and new guidelines they are supposed to follow. Compliance is low because they are rarely supplied with scientific evidence supporting a change in procedure, are rarely asked how this new idea might be best adapted to the daily routine of their particular unit, and rarely get feedback on whether it is improving care. By opening up these conversations, doctors and nurses not only have a better understanding of the reason for the change but also feel they are part of the process—that their opinion matters.

Just as with the placing of central lines, there are existing guidelines for many of the procedures we do every day in intensive care. However, these guidelines are similarly shrouded in often ambiguous, nonprioritized, and cryptic encyclopedia-size volumes that are not very helpful in the fast-paced clinical setting of the ICU. For central lines we condensed those guidelines into straightforward, simple, and concise checklists, overcame barriers, measured performance, and effectively reduced related infections.

Our success at virtually eliminating central line infections in the SICU created a spark. And we wanted to use this spark to ignite a wildfire of change throughout the hospital and health care—a fire whose light we hoped would illuminate the dim corners of hospital culture and expose bad systems that we were convinced were harming patients.

With this in mind we structured the TRIP model using four key principles:

1. Summarize evidence into checklists.
2. Identify and mitigate local barriers to implementation.
3. Measure performance.
4. Ensure all patients reliably receive the intervention.

These principles were applied as follows. Once we have identified a diagnosis, treatment, or procedure that is putting patients at risk, we put together an interdisciplinary team—physicians, nurses, researchers, technicians, and administrators—and create a checklist using evidence-based interventions that are the most effective at improving patient outcomes (the CDC guidelines and the U.S. government Web site www.guidelines.gov are great resources for this). We also incorporate what clinicians have learned firsthand on the unit. We try to select no more than seven items that have the greatest benefit, have the lowest risks and costs, and are easiest and most +/ practical for the unit to implement.

Next we identify any barriers that might prevent patients from receiving the items on the checklist. A barrier could be a clinician who is not aware of, or does not agree with, the items on the checklist. The checklist items may be ambiguous so the clinicians are unsure who is to do what and when. Or clinicians might have insufficient training and supervision to perform the checklist or lack the proper equipment. To help identify barriers, staff members are observed implementing the checklist. Team members should also "walk the process," actually performing items on the checklist. This illuminates additional problems that might have been invisible to an observer. We also encourage open discussions among staff about their thoughts on the checklist and why they think it might be difficult to use. When barriers are identified, the team should not just encourage clinicians to "try harder." Most likely they are already trying very hard. Instead they should make changes in the way work is being performed and organized that make it easier to comply with the checklist.

After this, we measure outcomes or performance and compare them with the baseline measures to see whether the checklist actually improves patient outcomes. The team will need to create data collection forms and a database. They will need to train staff to accurately collect the data, develop plans to track and identify missing data, and provide regular reports on their performance.

Measurement is one of the most important aspects of our work. We are scientists and the cornerstone of science is measurement. Without hard scientific proof, we can't be sure something actually works. Similarly, if we can't judge a theory's performance, how can we improve on it? It's like teaching a baseball pitcher how to throw on target while wearing a blindfold. If they can't see the results, they can't learn. Also, limited resources restrict the number of safety initiatives a hospital can adopt. Therefore, without knowing if an initiative is effective, how can a hospital be sure the investment is actually making patients safer? In addition, without complete and compelling data, it's hard to get doctors on board. This is both expected and appropriate. Doctors are scientists at heart, and as such they depend on real evidence, not guesswork. If we are asking physicians to change how they care for patients, those doctors need to be sure that patients are better off because of that change. And if doctors are not on board, the initiative is dead in the water. Finally, without accurate data we cannot be held accountable for our results. We cannot in good conscience tell the public, policy makers, the payers of health care, or patients that we have made health care safer. I'm both a physician and a trained researcher, and as such, if validly measured results do not support a theory, the theory is likely not true. (This regard for science has been sorely lacking in the majority of patient safety work.)

As I have already stated, there were significant advantages to experimenting with these theories in the ICU where I worked. I knew the layout and had some authority. But there is another good reason for choosing an ICU for our work—it's the canary in the coal mine for detecting errors. ICUs are one of the largest, most expensive, and complex components of the U.S. health care system. Errors here are more common, easier to detect, and have much more severe consequences. ICU patients are on the very precipice of death, making even the slightest mistake both immediate and striking.

Bloodstream infections are a perfect example. A relatively healthy person admitted to a regular inpatient unit might not develop a serious blood infection if a doctor forgets to wash his hands before inserting a central line. But imagine the same scenario with a kidney transplant patient in the ICU who is receiving medication that suppresses his immune system so his own body's defense system won't reject the kidney. If a nasty little bacterium enters his bloodstream, it can spread unchecked—and sometimes even kill him.

Despite the sense of urgency and level of intensity in the ICU, errors are common. One study concluded that there were 1.7 errors per patient per day in America's ICUs. Of these errors, 29 percent could have caused clinically significant harm or death. Given that the average ICU length of stay is three days, this research suggests that nearly all patients hospitalized in the ICU sustain a potentially life-threatening mistake at some point during their stay. That is a frightening statistic. That means that approximately 85,000 errors occur every day in ICUs across the country, and 24,650 of those are potentially life threatening.

Even more disturbing, these numbers reflect errors related to what doctors and nurses actively do wrong to patients. If we include things we should have done but failed to—for example, diagnostic errors in which we fail to give the correct therapy, delay the correct therapy, or give the wrong therapy, or neglecting to use sterile procedures when placing a central line—the number of deaths and complications due to errors increase dramatically.

That is not to say that ICUs are bad for patients. These units save many lives by providing life-saving support for failing bodies. Nevertheless, complex systems—of which ICUs are certainly an example—are breeding grounds for errors. Many physicians, nurses, and other staff care for ICU patients. Each of these clinicians uses highly sensitive and potentially dangerous technologies and medications. Yet many procedures are not standardized. Even if standards exist, the steps are not always followed. Communication between doctors and nurses is poor, leaving some members of the care team feeling isolated, and the plan of care is often not clear. Sometimes the treatments that one doctor prescribes to help the lungs might hurt the heart or kidneys. Unless there is a strong team effort to integrate these therapies and select the therapy with the most practical risk-benefit ratio for the entire body, patients can suffer. Such complex systems require careful planning and excellent teamwork and communication. Yet to date there are no generally accepted national or statewide standards for the majority of the procedures that occur daily in the ICU.

VAP

One life-threatening illnesses that is relatively common to the ICU is ventilator-associated pneumonia (VAP)—an infection that can occur with patients placed on mechanical ventilators (breathing machines). Like central line infections, this problem is for the most part preventable, making it an excellent pilot test for our newly formed TRIP model. To add another little challenge for our model, we decided to focus our research on the recently opened Weinberg ICU (WICU). Like the SICU, the WICU serves an accompanying suite of operating rooms. I worked as an attending physician in the WICU as well. This new facility provided intensive care for cancer patients who had undergone surgical treatments. Dr. Sean Berenholtz was also an attending physician on that unit. Sean, who holds a degree in clinical investigation and shares my passion for patient safety, helped lead our study on central line infections and VAPs.

In any ICU it is fairly common to place a patient on mechanical ventilation; sick patients often have difficulty breathing or cannot breathe at all on their own. Yet one of the dangers with mechanical ventilators is they are associated with high rates of pneumonia, resulting in higher costs and increased mortality.

We put together a TRIP team, studied the research on this procedure, and prepared a simple checklist that identified five key steps to prevent ventilator-associated pneumonia.

- *Elevate the head of the bed so that it is at or above 30 degrees.* This helps mucus from the mouth and nose drain into the stomach instead of the lungs.
- *Limit the sedation of patients so that they are able to follow commands at least once a day.* In the past most ventilated patients were kept asleep the entire time they were in the ICU. Clinicians thought it was safer and easier to keep patients out cold. But research has shown this is not true. In fact, the risk of pneumonia and other complications is greatly decreased if patients are kept awake.
- *Test every day whether the patient still needs the ventilator.* Every day a patient is on a breathing machine gives him a 1 to 3 percent chance of developing pneumonia; the longer you are on the ventilator the greater the risk.

Although not associated with pneumonia, we also included the following two steps on the checklist because evidence showed they improved the patient's general health when ventilated.

- *Provide medication for stomach ulcers.* A large number of patients on ventilation develop ulcers because of the stress ventilation puts on the body's systems.
- *Provide medication for blood clots.* Patients on ventilation do not move around as much and are at risk for developing a life-threatening blood clot in a deep vein, often in the leg (a condition called deep vein thrombosis).

Nobody disputed that each of these items on the checklist made sense and would potentially save lives. Yet, before we implemented TRIP, these interventions were followed inconsistently. In the WICU, for example, patients received all five of these procedures only 30 percent of the time. Interestingly enough, that was the same level of baseline compliance we saw with the central line checklist. (It seems this is the kind of performance health care delivers when processes are not standardized.)

So we educated clinicians about the evidence supporting the checklist, added it to our daily routine, and encouraged nurses, pharmacists, and respiratory therapists to watch physicians and make sure that patients received these therapies. We also had staff walk the process and observe and talk to their fellow clinicians to identify further potential barriers to compliance.

One of the barriers we identified was keeping the bed elevated at or above 30 degrees. There was no clear way of telling when the bed was situated correctly. So we put a gauge on the side of the bed. This not only gave clarity to the measure but it also worked to visually remind nurses and doctors because they saw that gauge every time they visited the patient.

Another barrier we found was both striking and sobering. We surveyed nurses and asked why they should do the items on the checklist. Nearly all the nurses responded, "Because the doctor ordered it." They did not say because patients will benefit from it or because there is strong evidence to support using it. Rather, the nurses saw themselves as simply following orders.

When we investigated this problem we found that the nurses on our unit had not been fully educated on the science behind the VAP checklist. Few understood or believed that these techniques were actually proven to lower infection rates. We stepped up our training and made sure nurses knew they were a valuable part of the research team and that they fully comprehended how the checklist made patients safer. Lightbulbs went on and compliance increased.

Another barrier we discovered was that the order to do the VAP checklist had to be initiated by a physician. If the physician forgot, the intervention would not be done and the necessary equipment would not be ordered. So we made it an automatic order for all patients entering the unit. This way all patients got the therapy unless a physician consciously decided the patients didn't need it. In addition, the necessary equipment would automatically get delivered to the unit.

Probably the most radical step we took to promote the checklist was that we gave it to family members of patients in the WICU. We explained how it worked and why it worked and encouraged these nonclinicians to observe and ask nurses and doctors if the procedures were being followed. This might sound as if it would interfere with patient care (we heard this very complaint from physicians and nurses alike), but in the end it was very successful. Many family members were in or around the ICU anyway and they often asked a lot of questions. Since they usually had limited knowledge of the care plan, many of these questions were superfluous and not effective at helping improve their loved ones' care. Now that family members were aware of the checklist, they were asking useful questions that actually helped the nurses and doctors do their jobs.

The education and reorganization of the work environment paid off handsomely. Compliance with the checklist improved to more than 95 percent. Unfortunately, we could not make a definitive conclusion about infection rates since VAPs have many different definitions and there is no consensus among experts. But studies have shown that compliance with the items on our checklist significantly reduces the number of ventilated patients who develop pneumonia, which, in turn, lowers the length of stay for these patients. This makes it possible to both accommodate additional patients and minimize the time that critical patients in the emergency department or operating room have to wait for a bed in the ICU.

Since it costs roughly twenty-two thousand dollars each time a patient in the ICU develops pneumonia, and as much as five thousand dollars for each additional day a patient stays in the ICU, this checklist not only potentially saves lives but also saves hospitals and patients a significant amount of money.

Thanks to our success with central lines and VAPs, word was spreading about our work. A new field of research was gaining attention and respect: patient safety research. This type of applied research traditionally received limited recognition or validation in academic medicine, primarily because of a lack of scientific methods. By applying real science to this kind of work, and measuring results, we are beginning to turn this around.

Our success also created momentum for our work at the hospital level. Nurses and doctors alike were attracted to both the science behind the work and the results. Health care is both emotionally and physically demanding. We suffer daily with little time to process our feelings, and we work long hours, often getting calls in the middle of the night, and are expected to be at the top of our game whenever needed. New ideas, even if they are designed to save time, initially create more work. It's always easier, in the short term, to do things the old way. However, we're in the business of saving lives and healing bodies and minds. All you have to do is prove to the doctors or nurses that a new initiative improves care, and they get on board, even if it means a little more work. Our success gave nurses and doctors that extra drive.

With this momentum behind us, we decided to expand our horizons beyond the ICU and tackle a problem that affected the operating room—surgical site infections (SSI). That's when we hit a roadblock.

SSIs are precisely what they sound like, infections that attack the parts of the body where a surgeon has made his incisions. SSIs cause anywhere from 300,000 to 1 million infections a year in American hospitals, significantly increasing the likelihood of death from a surgical procedure. And although these infections cause fewer deaths than either central lines or VAP, they are a significant national problem. Dr. Elizabeth Martinez, a colleague of mine in the Department of Anesthesiology and Critical Care Medicine who is trained in clinical investigation, helped lead this project. For this, just as we did with central line infections, we worked closely with our hospital epidemiology and infection control colleagues.

Just as they do for central line infections and VAPs, the CDC and other professional societies produce guidelines on how to prevent SSIs. And just like with these other diseases, we needed to condense these guidelines into a checklist that would highlight the most important interventions in the guideline and summarize them. When we started, we had no clue how often doctors and nurses followed the required procedures that were known to prevent these infections, but brief observation and experience suggested it was not often. We also did not know the barriers to using them. Using the TRIP model, we formed a team to explore the problem and created our first checklist:

- Avoid shaving the patient.
- Keep the patient warm.
- Provide antibiotics on time.
- Readminister or redose antibiotics at correct time intervals.
- Control the patient's blood sugar level.

As expected, we found barriers to doing these steps. One of these was that staff had a hard time remembering what antibiotic to give for each specific operation and how often the antibiotic needed to be redosed. The antibiotic recommended to prevent SSIs varies by the type of surgery and whether the patient has an allergy to penicillin, which many do. Doctors need to remember hundreds of antibiotic/ surgery combinations. In addition, each antibiotic has a different dosing interval. Some antibiotics are given every four hours, some every six, some every eight, others every twelve or twenty-four hours. If a patient has kidney dysfunction these intervals can change. This one simple step to a safe operation requires doctors to remember hundreds of pieces of data, which they often forget, and, as a result, patients suffer.

We changed this. We worked with our colleagues in hospital epidemiology and infectious diseases and made a poster-size chart matching each type of surgery and the recommended antibiotic. We also standardized when patients needed to be redosed. But we still needed a system to ensure that patients received the additional dosing at the appropriate times. So we made a second chart clearly outlining the times when the next dose was due. We also standard-ized what antibiotics to give to patients with renal dysfunction and penicillin allergies.

Another problem with antibiotic dosing was that it was unclear whose responsibility it was—the surgeon's or the anesthesiologist's. We settled that ambiguity and assigned it to anesthesiologists. As expected, we got some resistance from some members of that de-partment, who believed it should be the responsibility of surgeons. However, with strong support from the department chairman, John Ulatowski, and the persistence of Elizabeth, the anesthesiologists eventually recognized this as an opportunity and embraced it.

After addressing these and other barriers, it seemed like we were in good shape. Everyone on the team felt that we had caught most of the problems and fixed them. Naturally we expected good results. After all, surgical site infections couldn't be much harder to tackle than bloodstream infections. What we didn't anticipate, however, were the complex cultural dynamics we would face stepping into the often-intense arena of the operating room, where most of these infections originate.

The operating room is one of the most complex places in the hospital, emotionally, socially, and politically, where high-stakes, high-anxiety procedures are the norm. Anesthesiologists give patients medications that make them lifeless and stop their breathing. If the anesthesiologist does not correctly put in a breathing tube, in the right place, so a ventilator can breathe for the patient, the patient will die. When the surgeon cuts into the patient's body, the anxiety only amplifies. One wrong move of the scalpel can result in catastrophic hemorrhage. Not surprisingly, emotions are elevated; conflicts are common and tantrums—little different from those of a toddler—are almost daily occurrences.

The political structure within the operating room is also complicated. There are scores of discipline-specific teams (anesthesiologists, nurses, surgeons) and procedure-specific teams (neurosurgery, cardiac surgery, urology, gynecology), as well as subteams and cliques within each group. This complex team structure makes it incredibly difficult to convey messages and safety programs throughout the entire operating room. When messages are communicated, it's like playing the telephone game: the message delivered is often strikingly different from the message received.

Operating rooms are also exceedingly hierarchical. They have a pecking order that is stronger and stricter than the marines. The operating room is a world of ritual and privilege, a world of special favors for the elite.

For example, when we don't have an available bed in the ICU, sometimes we need to cancel a surgical case that will need an ICU bed after surgery. It would be unsafe and unethical to do otherwise. We have developed a fair and logical decision tree for which cases will be canceled. However, if an intensivist, like me, follows this established system and cancels a surgery because of a shortage of beds in the ICU, a few of the surgical attendings will likely go ballistic and exercise all his rather extensive influence and muscle to change the order. While most surgeons behave appropriately; some predictably do not. So, to avoid this unpleasant outburst, these cases are never canceled. Is this just or even safe? Absolutely not. Is it politically wise for hospital staff? Yes. And so it continues.

Many of these types of scenarios are permitted because experienced surgeons are hard to replace. They are highly valued by the institution (primarily because they bring in a lot of revenue) and therefore protected. But it does not foster teamwork or goodwill and it puts patients at risk. Yet it continues, mostly because it stems from long-standing hierarchical culture.

Our first big challenge with reducing SSIs was getting surgeons to stop shaving the surgical site. Surgeons mistakenly believed that shaving actually lowers, rather than increases, infection risks. We had numerous group discussions about this, shared the evidence and the stories, but the surgeons kept doing it their way. We even removed all the razors from the operating room, stopped ordering them, and replaced them with clippers—shown to lower infection risks. Yet surgeons would not give in. Some actually hid razors in secret places and smuggled them into the operating room. It was bizarre. Yet in a strange way, it was rational. The surgeons are strong advocates for their patients and they want to do what they can to reduce a patient's risk for complications, including SSIs. They wrongly believed that shaving lowered infection risk. This belief was based on information more than a decade old but also on their direct observation—when they used a razor they got a clean shave; when they used the clippers, some hairs remained and, theoretically, could fall into the wound. Surgeons reasoned, wrongly, that clean-shaved skin would have a lower infection risk than skin with stubble. If these doctors had a way to monitor their own infection rates they would have known this assumption was wrong. Or if they had read the studies, published mostly in medical and infectious disease journals, they would have realized their assumptions were wrong. But some of these surgeons either were not listening to or were not trusting the wisdom of other experts. So they continued to believe that smooth skin was safer than stubble. Yet research has proven that shaving causes injury to the skin, creating many tiny cuts that break down the immune barrier that skin provides, therefore increasing infection risks.

Yet surgeons continued to resist. They hid razors in their offices and conspired with nurses—some of whom also thought smoothly shaved skin was safer and some of whom did not want to upset the surgeons. These nurses would hide razors in their lockers and retrieve them when the surgeon requested. We had a black market for razors and the price was high.

This problem, like so many, was purely cultural. The surgeons had their beliefs, and we couldn't get them to change their view. Until we found a way to convince them that the patients would benefit from not being shaved, they would continue to use razors.

One easy and rather inaccurate assumption one could make here is that people, generally, resist change. But it's not change alone that they find troubling. If a person inherited $60 million, it would likely change his or her life; I know it would change mine. Yet few, if anyone would say, "No, keep the money; I hate change." People don't fear change, they fear loss. And loss has two components, a real component and a perceived component, and the perceived is generally larger and more powerful. Yet it is often unproven, generally false, and grossly exaggerated. What leaders of change need to do is minimize real losses and demonstrate that perceived losses are mythical. Only then can they successfully implement change.

In addition to the surgeons' refusal to abandon their razors, cultural divisions started to rear their ugly heads. Tensions started to build between anesthesiologists, nurses, and surgeons, each blaming the other for the high infection rate. Nurses and anesthesiologists were saying, "Surgeons are arrogant, they're not team players." Surgeons were saying, "Those nurses are incompetent. They never have the equipment I need. They're slow getting the OR ready for the next surgery. Nobody but me cares about the patients." Surgeons also complained that anesthesiologists were lazy, didn't care, and didn't work with the team to get patients in and out of the operating room efficiently.

Our previous work in the SICU and WICU was successful because the team was united; we worked together all the time. Yet the operating room team was a team in name only. In fact the surgeons are the only real core; the anesthesiologists and nurses shift around, based on need. While this may be more efficient and cost-effective for the hospital, it is not necessarily good for patients or staff, who clearly benefit from consistent teams that learn to work well together. People who work together in the operating room are often strangers who don't even know each other's names. As a result, these "teams" are generally more confrontational than cooperative, more independent than interdependent. Interestingly, nurses almost always know the names of the surgeon and anesthesiologist. (In fact they often know their first names yet are afraid to use them.) Conversely, surgeons and anesthesiologists often do not know the nurses' first or last names. This ancient custom only further exacerbates the cultural divides. Aviation learned this lesson the hard way. Studies that examined airline accidents and crew configurations revealed that in 75 percent of accidents the pilot and copilot had never flown together. Not being familiar with team members is perilous in the sky and in health care.

With this complex organizational structure, it proved exceedingly difficult to get everyone engaged in the TRIP model. As a result, we didn't reduce infection rates like we had hoped to.

In hindsight, I am not surprised we failed to permeate the culture inside the operating room. I'm an anesthesiologist so I understand this world. I live it. Perhaps it's the immediate life-or-death urgency that exists in that arena. Perhaps it's the fact that surgeons are almost required to rule autonomously, and therefore often possess unyielding egos. Perhaps they need this level of confidence to cut into someone's brain, heart, or intestines. Whatever the case, the culture in the operating room is thick and often toxic. At its worst, it resembles the kind of name-calling and immaturity you might see in a middle school playground.

Once, I was administering anesthesia to a patient in the operating room who was having surgery for a recurrent ventral hernia. This is a gap in the muscles of the abdominal wall, in her case near her belly button, which causes an unsightly bulging. Ventral hernias are often painful and potentially life threatening.

An hour and a half into the surgery her blood pressure dropped, her face turned red, and she began wheezing and having difficulty breathing. These are the classic symptoms of an allergic reaction. I quickly reviewed the medicines we had given her. She was not allergic to any of them so I suspected she was suffering from a latex allergy. She had undergone ten previous operations, and this type of allergy is common among patients who have undergone multiple surgeries. (In fact, today we no longer use any form of latex anywhere in the hospital, to avoid this very complication.)

Surgical latex allergies are often severe, due to the direct exposure of the allergen to the patient's blood supply. They can easily lead to anaphylactic shock and death in a matter of minutes, and without treatment they are deadly. This was exactly what was happening to this patient. Realizing this, I gave her epinephrine, the drug you use to treat this condition. Her symptoms went away immediately.

I told the surgeon that I thought the patient was experiencing a latex allergy and recommended that he change his gloves to a non-latex variety we also stocked in the operating room. The surgeon responded, "You're wrong. This can't be a latex allergy. We have been operating for an hour and a half and the patient didn't experience a reaction to latex during any of her previous procedures."

I replied, "I am fairly certain this is a latex allergy. Latex allergies often develop after a patient, like this one, has had multiple surgeries and they can start anytime during the case. You just got into her abdomen and the latex only recently came in contact with her blood, which is why we didn't see the reaction before. You need to change your gloves to reduce further latex exposure. If she stays stable, you can finish the operation."

In the meantime the patient's symptoms returned—epinephrine only lasts for a few minutes. I gave her another dose and the symptoms went away again. At this point there was no doubt in my mind that she had a latex allergy. So I asked the surgeon, again, to change his gloves. But the surgeon refused.

He said, "There is no way this is a latex allergy and I am not changing my gloves, now let me finish the operation; that is why we are all here."

"Let's think through this situation," I said. "If I'm wrong, then you will waste five minutes changing gloves. If you are wrong, the patient dies. Do you really think this risk-benefit ratio warrants you not changing your gloves?" see p. 34

I thought this clearly would convince the surgeon to change his gloves, but instead the surgeon hunkered down further and said again, "You're wrong, this is clearly not an allergic reaction, so I'm not changing my gloves."

I responded, "How confident are you that this is not a latex allergy? What else do you think could be causing her problems?"

The resident standing next to me was ashen and the nurses were speechless. Honestly, in this situation, most anesthesiologists would cower. (I certainly have in the past.) These types of conflicts occur daily in hospitals and surgical teams are poor at resolving them. This is understandable because the staff receives little to no training in conflict management despite the fact that conflict is a common, costly, and often lethal problem. The way most of these conflicts are resolved is the surgeon exercises his authority, as was the case here. In the operating room the surgeon is the captain of the ship. What he says goes, even if the issue, as in this case, is something for which he is not the expert. This patient was experiencing a medical, not a surgical, problem. I was far more qualified to make this call.

I couldn't let this patient die just because the surgeon didn't want to change gloves. But to be honest, I was not quite sure what do to. I had trained in conflict management and had already used the tools I had learned. But I hadn't made much of an impact on this surgeon. The patient's blood pressure continued to drop dangerously, her wheezing returned, and her blood oxygen was low. If we did not reduce her exposure to latex quickly, she would die. Since reasoning did not work, I needed to pull rank and go up the chain of command. I needed to get an authority figure to command this surgeon to change his gloves. By now I was a respected safety leader in the hospital, and I was confident that senior hospital leaders would not tolerate his behavior and would support me. But how could I reach them quickly? There was little time to spare and I was in the operating room, giving epinephrine, trying to save a dying patient. I told the surgeon his answer was unacceptable. I said loudly to the nurse, "Please 'stat' page Dean Miller and Mr. Peterson, the hospital president."

I told the surgeon that I could guarantee that the administrators would not find it acceptable to put the patient and the institution at risk in this way. The nurse walked over to the phone, picked it up, and looked up at me. Nobody had asked her to do this before. The surgeon's orders are never challenged. The nurse paused and I said, "Page them now. This patient is having a latex allergy. I cannot let her die because we did not change gloves." The nurse started to dial. The surgeon said an expletive, dropped his gloves, and went out to change them.

After the surgery, tests confirmed that the patient was allergic to latex. If I had not acted, the consequences could have been catastrophic. This patient could have died from ignorance and arrogance—a lethal combination. With the exhaustive volume of medical knowledge out there, doctors can't be expected to know everything. That's why they have to work with the team and be humble enough to listen to the advice of their teammates. The ignorance was understandable; the arrogance was not. This gross lack of communication, respect, cooperation, and teamwork, in the end, harms everyone—patients, doctors, and nurses alike.

In this particular case, the patient was fortunate because I was already gaining a reputation and support inside Hopkins as a safety leader. That gave me the courage to speak up because I believed the dean and president of the hospital would most likely back me up. What if I was just starting out in my career? What if I did not know these senior leaders personally? Would I have taken such a risk, breaking the chain of command and challenging a surgeon? Perhaps not. If the patient had died, it would have been blamed primarily on her allergy, not the surgeon. Similar dramas play out day after day in hospitals across the country. How many patients have been harmed or died as a result? Will we ever really know?

It is important to note that this was the first time I had worked with this particular surgeon. The two surgeons I normally worked with on these operations would have changed their gloves if asked. This is most likely because we had an established working relationship, which provided a strong platform for good communication and teamwork. But many surgical teams have not worked together, and might not trust or respect each other's judgment or skill, opening the door for hazardous scenarios like the one that almost killed our patient.

Everyone would agree this is unacceptable. Yet there is no system in place that addresses culture and teamwork in the operating room, or in any part of the hospital for that matter. And bad culture exists throughout medicine. And it's not only doctors who are to blame. Poor communication and lousy teamwork are a problem in every level of health care, from administrative assistants to top executives. No person or department is immune to this problem.

The reason we had success with our programs in the ICU was because we had a leg up on culture. The ICU was our workplace and we had already established strong relationships with the staff. With SSIs we were addressing culture in someone else's domain, in this case the operating room, which notoriously has an intense culture dynamic.

It is also important to note that bad culture is not confined to Hopkins; it exists in all hospitals. We obtained a grant to develop the SSI program at five academic medical institutions across the Northeast. Yet before we could even launch the study, cultural barriers surfaced. At the start of the project, we had a meeting with surgery, anesthesia, and nursing leaders from all the institutions participating in the study. They agreed to support efforts to reduce SSIs as long as it didn't increase their workload or require that they collect data. Others were willing to implement the checklist but didn't want to address culture. In essence, most of the hospitals we were planning to work with wanted to control these efforts so it would have the least impact on the staff. They wanted a quick hit, an easy and painless change. But I had learned that there is no easy way to make hospitals safer; it requires hard work and the willingness to change age-old cultural patterns. Without that commitment, it just won't work.

One of key components of TRIP is to identify procedures that have the highest benefit to the patients and condense them into a checklist. However, what we ultimately learned was that to ensure that patients actually received these improvements, a cultural change was required. Good culture is the lubrication that allows us to redesign systems—without it, sparks fly. TRIP had a culture component, but it was not strong enough to overcome the resistance we faced outside of the ICU. I knew if my team and I were going to successfully expand this to other units, we would have to come up with a separate tool—a tool whose primary focus was to improve teamwork and culture.

So I gathered my team, pulled out the drawing board, and headed back to the ICU to develop what would become our second model, the comprehensive unit-based safety program (CUSP). This program would focus primarily on building teamwork and improving culture in the unit, with the hope that this would create a platform on which change would be not only possible but successful. It turned out to be just what we needed.

*CUSP.*

# Chapter 4

C ulture is local. It occurs in the cracks and corners of hospitals and is unique to each and every unit. Indeed, studies have shown that variations in culture between units in a hospital are four times greater than the variations in culture between hospitals. Listen to the stories in the break rooms or how doctors and nurses talk during rounds—the culture is palpable. What we needed was a program that focused primarily on this local culture, a program that worked at the unit level to help train physicians, nurses, and other staff to work together effectively as a team. We needed a program that could be used in all units in the hospital yet was flexible enough to address each unit's unique risks.

As I have already demonstrated, the operating room teaches us a lot about hospital culture. It's a tense environment where ego, autonomy and competition often make it difficult to build good teamwork and communication. Surgeons generally run the operating room with supreme authority, which in some ways is understandable and necessary. In a critical life-or-death environment like this, someone has to be in charge. If and when things go south, the team needs to act fast and act definitively and someone has to be calling the shots. There is no time for a vote, no time to argue about plan of action.

Yet in other hierarchical industries, like the military, the organization is rapidly able to level that hierarchy in risky situations. For example, on an aircraft carrier, a person who is sweeping the deck can wave off a plane if the landing area has debris that could pose risks for a crash. The deckhands are not penalized for taking this action; they are rewarded. Most complex industries recognize that teams make wise decisions with diverse and independent input; in fact, they encourage it. Yet in medicine, we have not learned this. When I saw impending disaster—a patient about to die from a latex allergy—I told my surgeon to change his course, but he totally dismissed my warnings. What makes this even more disturbing is the surgeon and I are more alike, in training, than the pilot and his deckhand—we both went to medical school, we both did residencies. In fact, as an anesthesiologist and critical care specialist, I was likely more qualified to make this call. Yet, my warnings were still dismissed. This is unacceptable. Surgeons, and for that matter all doctors, must learn to release some authority and open their minds to other possible solution and explanations. What I was saying to this surgeon made sense, and even if I was wrong, a good leader would have seen the risk-benefit ratio and acted accordingly. Yet the surgeon decided not to change course.

Our safety team reviewed the liability claims and errors that resulted in substantial harm to patients at a number of hospitals, and in nearly 90 percent of these events, one of the care team members knew something was wrong and either kept silent or spoke up but was ignored. Patients pay an awfully high price for dysfunctional teamwork.

This is another example where medicine can learn from aviation. Forty years ago, most accidents in aviation were the result of mechanical failures, usually due to the unreliability of the piston engine. However, after 1971, when the turbine engine became the norm for most commercial aircraft, the blame shifted to pilot error—specifically communication between pilots and copilots in the cockpit.

In January 1982, Air Florida Flight 90 crashed into the Fourteenth Street Bridge on the Potomac River in Washington, D.C. The accident happened in a severe snowstorm immediately after the jet took off from Washington National Airport in Virginia, killing seventy passengers, four crew members, and four motorists on the bridge. Only five people on the plane survived. The nightly news showed graphic pictures of passengers being plucked from the icy Potomac River by firefighters.

The accident was blamed on a number of errors—notably the crew's failure to properly deice the wings before takeoff, and its decision to proceed with takeoff, in spite of iced wings. But one error really grabbed the attention of airline safety officials. As the plane started to lift off, the first officer did not think they had enough power for a successful takeoff. He repeatedly voiced his concern, but the captain chose to ignore these warnings.

It was later confirmed that they had plenty of runway left to abort takeoff. It is conceivably understandable that the pilots might have misjudged the level of icing on the wings and misjudged the real danger. However, the fact that the pilot chose to completely ignore the warnings of his chief officer is totally unacceptable. Like so many autonomous doctors, the pilot decided not to listen to his most trusted adviser, his copilot.

The investigation of this tragedy prompted a study into the way pilots and copilots interact in the cockpit. After a series of simulator tests it soon became very apparent that pilots, for the most part, don't listen to copilots. This is terrifyingly similar to the culture in

the operating room, where the chief surgeon is the captain and almost everyone else in the room is a copilot. And just as the cockpit
is the most critical area in a plane, there are few places in a hospital
where culture has more of an enormous and immediate impact on
safety and outcomes of patients than the operating room. A mistake there can kill, and very quickly. Given the level of urgency,
one would expect this unit to function with the precision and efficiency of a Swiss clock. Yet many surgical teams don't even know the
names or roles of their colleagues, even after working together for
years. I remember speaking to a nurse who had been working with a
surgeon for two decades. The surgeon had just left the room and she
had tears in her eyes. I asked her what was the matter and if I could
help. She said, "I have worked for twenty years with him, I have bent
over backward to make this place work and his life better, and he
does not even know my name."

Many surgeons are aware of the toxic culture in the operating
room and how it could potentially harm patients. General surgeon
Martin Makary, recalls his experiences working in the Hopkins
trauma operating room as a resident. "We were all wearing the same
green pajamas and nobody was introduced; there was just a lot of
yelling, 'Hey, you, give me this or do that.' Often I didn't know if I
was talking with a technician or the chief of surgery."

With this level of cultural ambiguity, errors are frequent. One
of those errors—not only common but especially terrifying and
repugnant—is wrong-site surgery. This happens when a surgeon
mistakenly operates on the wrong part of the body, usually the wrong
side of the body—such as removing the wrong kidney or amputat-
ing the right arm instead of the left arm or the left breast instead of
the right. It's estimated that there are close to four thousand wrong-
site surgeries every year in American hospitals. Sometimes names

are confused and we even operate on the wrong patient—someone who is supposed to have his kidney removed might lose his pancreas instead.

For years, incidences of wrong-site surgery were kept hidden from the press and public and often from other clinicians for obvious reasons of liability and reputation. During my residency I had a patient with a broken ankle that needed surgery. I was assigned to place an "ankle block," a procedure in which I was to inject local anesthetic into several nerves around the ankle to make it numb so that the painful procedure could be performed. The consent form said the surgery was on the left ankle, yet it turned out to be the right ankle that was broken. Luckily I spoke to the patient and discovered the error and placed the block on the correct side. If I had just blindly followed the consent form (as many do) and numbed the left side, I would have had to go back and numb the right side. That would have meant that after the operation the patient would not have been able to walk and would have had to be hospitalized—incurring more cost and causing him more discomfort.

At that time, wrong-site surgery was not viewed as a significant problem. We did not have formal error reporting systems—so there was no report of my event and no investigation. In essence, the institution did not take steps to learn how to avoid the mistake in the future. I felt troubled about it, but that was about all that happened.

Wrong-site surgery gained public attention in 1995 when the press got hold of a story about a patient at the University Community Hospital in Tampa, Florida, who had the wrong leg amputated. This event unleashed a flood of previously unreported cases, prompting the Joint Commission (a nonprofit organization that regulates hospital standards and safety) to study the issue. The commission subsequently issued a mandate requiring all operating room teams perform a "time-out" before every surgical procedure to ensure the surgeons had the right patient, the right procedure, and the right surgical site.

The time-out requires that surgeons literally mark the surgical site preoperatively. It also states that before any incision is made, operating nurses and physicians collectively review the case, the name of the patient, and the nature of the procedure. This ensures everyone is clear on exactly what is supposed to be done and if there are any questions or concerns, members of the team are encouraged to speak up.

Although the protocol makes sense and is necessary, it is based on a relatively limited understanding of the causes of the problem, one of which is culture. Furthermore, it wasn't tested first to see whether the intervention works. Patients were being harmed, so the Joint Commission wanted to act fast. Hope got in the way of science and time-outs were quickly introduced throughout the United States as mandatory. No doubt this is a tough balancing act, yet the "shoot first, ask questions later" approach to safety has had little impact on reducing patient harm.

Just as one might expect, many surgeons in operating rooms across the country dismiss the time-out as a perfunctory nuisance, and some even openly mock it. Surprisingly, since the regulation was put in place, reports of wrong-site surgery have actually increased. Although most of this is due to an increase in reporting, almost everyone agrees that the time-out is not as effective as it should be. And so the problem persists. The time-out is a checklist of sorts, and like all checklists, without culture change, they often don't work.

Martin clearly remembers the futility of the time-out at Hopkins. "When we did time-outs, we saw them as just another bureaucratic nuisance and no one took interest. Traditionally nurses would be off in the corner reading off the details of the procedure and maybe one person would respond. The problem is, when you do your residency for surgery you are told repeatedly that surgeons are above all other doctors and staff in the hospital. We have the longest, most rigorous, and most thorough training. It's as if we are trained not to listen to anyone else, not even the Joint Commission."

As we have said before, dysfunctional culture and poor teamwork exist in all areas of a hospital (and in fact they plague the entire national health care system). Early on in the WICU, when we were studying culture and its effect on care, we were trying to get clinicians to be aware when their workload exceeded a safe threshold. My goal was to better manage the demands on the entire team and make sure our patients were safely cared for at all times. When clinicians get overwhelmed, the likelihood of patient harm increases significantly. The problem is no one is willing to say his or her workload is too high. In hospitals there is a "suck it up" mentality, where a badge of courage is given to those who can do an incredible volume of work without complaining.

To better manage the workload and, in turn, make their hospital stay safer for patients, we convinced staff to wear colored cards that indicated the level of their load. Green meant "my workload is adequate, I have time to help someone whose load is excessive"; yellow meant "my workload is adequate, but I am at my limit and I can't help anyone"; and red meant "my workload is too high; I'm overwhelmed."

One day the ICU was full and we got two more patients from the emergency department. Both patients were in septic shock and dying. A third patient came from the operating room ahead of schedule and was bleeding badly—roughly a liter an hour—and needed to be resuscitated. Staff moved to help with this patient, leaving a

fourth patient unattended. This fourth patient stood up in a deliri-
ous, semiconscious state and quickly fell to the floor. Within a few
minutes our unit was in chaos. In the midst of all this, we got a call
from the operating room telling us they were bringing in yet another
patient. The charge nurse came running up to me and said, "Peter, I
am red, I am red."

I told her to call the operating room and tell them to keep that
patient until our workload went down. The nurse looked at me pan-
icked and said, "Peter, I can't do that, the hospital won't support
me."

In that moment, culture hit reality.

I asked, "What do you mean the hospital won't support you?"

The nurse responded, "If I do this, the surgeon, the nurse, and
the anesthesiologist will come running out of the OR screaming at
me, telling me that I am delaying the day and costing them money.
The hospital administration won't back me up."

"We have no choice," I told her. "The unit is in chaos right now
and we can't physically manage another patient. I'll take the heat.
Call them and have them hold their patient."

Culture, though always present, often becomes blatantly visible in times of stress. In spite of all our work on improving teamwork and communication in the WICU, the charge nurse, who is a
very good nurse, didn't believe that the institution would put safety
ahead of hospital business. She thought the institution only cared
about moving patients through, and that if she advocated for safety,
she would not be supported.

She was prescient. Sure enough, after she told the operating
room to hold the patient the surgeon came running over, red in the
face and screaming at her, "What are you doing? We can't leave that
patient in the operating room, I have another case to do."

I stepped in and politely told the surgeon, "We are doing what we can do. It is unsafe to take him in here. He'll have to stay in the operating room until our load lessens."

Similarly the surgical nurse came out of the operating room, annoyed, and said, "We're busy; we can't keep him."

As if on cue, the anesthesiologist came over, most likely thinking that since we were in the same department he might have more influence. "Peter, do you know what you are doing to the day's work?"

I addressed everybody and said in a calm voice, "I understand that very well. The workload is too high here and it is not safe. When it is lower we'll take him. If the patient was your mother, would you take her from an area where she could be adequately cared for to one in which she could not? We would be placing this patient in substantial danger if we took him, and that would not be fair to the patient or the staff."

The surgeon called hospital administration; the director of nursing asked to speak to me. She said, "Peter, what's going on down there? Why aren't you taking these patients? It's costing the hospital a lot of money."

I replied, "Thank you, but it's unsafe. The patient will stay in the operating room."

At the time it was exceedingly rare to halt scheduled surgeries because of a safety concern. But the reality is that there are times when a department's workload is so high it simply can't proceed. Every other industry limits the workload before it can exceed a safe capacity, yet this is strangely lacking in health care.

Once again, I had leverage because I had established a reputation as a leader in our institution's struggle to improve patient safety. I had the support of some very powerful administrators, including my department chair, the chair of surgery, the president of the hospital, and the dean of the medical school. In addition, the university president was a physician and exceedingly supportive of the work to improve safety. Without that kind of support, most physicians would be reluctant to put their head in the noose. The fault does not lie with health care workers but with the culture and systems in which they work. Yet, without a method in place that gives people confidence that their voice will be heard, culture cannot and will not change.

Changing the system is not just about changing the work process. It's not enough just to have a good idea (like asking surgeons not to shave patients because it increases infection rates), nor does it help just to work harder. We have to change the culture surrounding our work. We have to learn how we work better as a team. That will make the biggest dent in these safety issues. That much was clear to me.

There are countless examples of bad culture from every hospital across the nation. And even though we know bad culture can have a negative effect on patient care, it is rarely addressed, especially when it involves a physician. In fact, there are countless stories of hospitals protecting doctors who have seriously stepped out of line, even settling lawsuits just to keep the bad culture under wraps. A member of my safety team who worked for years as a nurse once summed it up well, saying, "If two doctors had a fistfight in the hall in front of patients and families, the most that would likely happen is the doctors would be talked to by their department chairs. However, if two nurses started swinging at each other, it is likely neither would have a job at the end of the day." Some of this might make sense from an administrative perspective since doctors pull in the most money, especially doctors that do procedures. However, this double standard hurts hospital culture, decreases productivity, and puts patients at risk.

Nurse researchers Deborah Dang, Dorothy Nyberg, and Jo Walrath are currently conducting a study to examine disruptive behavior in hospitals. Their preliminary findings, based on focus groups involving nurses, give great insights into the ways disruptive behavior, the cultural dynamics of teamwork and patient care, and safety interrelate.

Although the study focused primarily on how nurses experience these issues, it revealed culture issues across the spectrum of staff. The following are some examples of disruptive behavior that nurses reported.

"A resident will not listen or will not respond to a patient care concern. But, as I moved up the chain of command, I experienced consequences. After the attending spoke to the resident, the resident confronted me publicly for reporting her. Her profanity and body language were very threatening. My heart was racing, my hands were shaking. . . . I was scared for my safety," said one nurse in the study.

Another nurse talked about the abundance of disruptive non-verbal communication that occurs between doctors and nurses on the floor. "Turning your back to somebody when they are speaking to you, not making direct eye contact, shrugging things off . . . it interferes with care because if a physician shrugs you off when you are trying to report an abnormal finding, the next time you are going to think twice before you put yourself out there to be put down or humiliated."

Similarly, another nurse talked about being routinely ignored by doctors. "A nurse is concerned about a patient and calls the physician and tells him her concerns and assessment of the patient. The physician blows her off and does not attend to the patient. Then the nurse has to go up the chain of command to get someone who will come and see the patient and attend to their needs, which distracts the nurse from her patients. . . . And more importantly, the nurse learns to work around this physician and advises her colleagues to do the same."

Another nurse reported, "I made a simple but important point during patient rounds and I got yelled at in the middle of the unit in front of my patient and family members, which brought me to tears in a public forum. You can't imagine how humiliated I was."

These stories of misbehavior were not limited to doctors; they also happened when nurses were dealing with support staff.

"I dread making calls to the pharmacy or materials management for the fourth time for something that was stat and due an hour ago. They see these requests as a nurse's need and not a patient's need. . . .It is very frustrating. It is disruptive when the ancillary services don't remember or understand that we are all here for the patient and it's not a nursing need," said one of the nurses in the study.

Another nurse talked about the general miscommunication between all staff on the floor. "Things that are most disruptive in the workplace are the everyday rudeness. . . . It doesn't matter who it is—a physician, a nurse, an ancillary staff member—if it is a discourteous tone, it is very hard for me to get out of that state of emotion to think about something else for a while. . . . It affects your morale, your investment, how long you are willing to work, whether you feel like coming to work. When we are rude to each other it makes our jobs even harder."

These focus groups also revealed disruptive behavior between nurses on the floor, especially between senior and junior nurses. Just like everywhere in the hospital, there is a pecking order and it is not uncommon for junior nurses to be humiliated and berated by senior nurses, which directly affects morale and patient care.

"Younger, newer nurses need to be nurtured and mentored and are intimidated when the experienced nurse is sometimes very abrasive and direct," said one nurse.

Another nurse said this often-caustic environment creates such a negative work atmosphere that many new nurses have been literally driven from the hospital.

"Gossiping is quite maligning, very vindictive. People want to leave and run for the hills because of the intensity of the gossiping on a nursing unit," reported one nurse.

The hospital is a stressful environment to work in. Many clinicians are sleep deprived and overworked and they have little or no training in dealing with stress and conflict. In fact, in many ways the "suck it up" culture that is typical to medicine trains clinicians to deny these feelings. Without a system in place to help improve communication and teamwork among these hardworking individuals, it is both understandable and predictable that we see these kinds of disruptive behavior.

Poor communication does not always manifest itself in conflict, but it almost always erodes patient care. A patient came into one of the neurology rehabilitation units after having a cancerous tumor removed from his brain. He was developing a fever so the physician in charge of his case ordered blood to be drawn and sent to the lab to check for bloodstream infection. It was a Friday and the results did not come back in time for the weekday staff to read them. However, nobody on the regular staff notified the on-call weekend staff that this patient's tests needed to be checked and that he may be developing a bloodstream infection. To make things more complicated, in this unit the on-call physicians were brought in from a different hospital, so they did not have as much familiarity with the patients. The doctors came and did cursory rounds but did not make themselves aware of this patient's life-threatening condition and the need to check his lab results. There was no system in place to catch this error—to make sure this handoff between teams was performed efficiently and accurately. It was a standard example of poor communication, bad teamwork, and broken systems. When the weekday staff returned they found the man had a temperature of 103 degrees, was going into seizures, and had septic shock. A rapid-response team was called and the patient was sent to the neurosciences critical care unit and straight into surgery. This breakdown in communication and teamwork almost killed him.

It's clear that whether in the operating room, the ICU, a neurology unit, or anywhere teams have to work together to care for patients, bad culture, communication, and teamwork have a negative effect on that care. Our new comprehensive unit-based safety program (CUSP) would have to somehow address this culture and improve teamwork and communication if we were going to successfully improve safety. With this goal in mind we designed CUSP to focus on our most basic team structure—the work unit, where culture lives.            *CUSP*

A unit is a distinct group of doctors, nurses, technicians, and related staff who are clustered in a specific geography of the hospital and who often focus on a specific area of care. For example, the WICU is a sixteen-bed unit for cancer patients who have just undergone surgery. Patients are treated by a combination of intensivists, surgeons, critical care fellows, and surgery and anesthesiology residents. Similarly, Nelson-7 is an intermediate care nursing unit staffed by transplant surgeons, kidney and liver doctors whose focus is to get transplant recipients healthy enough to go home. Likewise, the operating room is a unit staffed by anesthesiologists and a variety of surgeons. Each of these units also contains an assortment of nurse practitioners, physician assistants, nurses, pharmacists, respiratory therapists, nutritionists, physical and occupational therapists, speech and language therapists, and social workers—clearly a complex and dynamic team.

The unit is where patient meets hospital, making it an obvious focal point for patient safety initiatives. Furthermore, by improving culture in the unit, we would in turn improve the way units interacted. That way, as patients moved through the hospital we would be better able to guarantee that they received high-quality care throughout their experience. We looked at units as building blocks. If we made these blocks strong, we could use them to build strong bridges between units and in turn make the entire hospital safe— from admission to discharge to outpatient care. But first we needed to create strong building blocks.

The goal of CUSP is to improve communication, teamwork, and culture in these individual units so they can focus more efficiently on the primary goal, improving patient outcomes.

We don't pick a problem, such as bloodstream infections, and then tell a unit to fix it. Instead, we ask the unit members to look around the workplace and identify safety issues they think need addressing. Specifically, we ask, "How do you think the next patient might be harmed?" and, "What can you do to prevent it?"

Usually you don't have to ask twice. Most people know exactly what in their work environment needs improving. Evidence has shown that in most industries, when workers think something is risky, it usually is. The problem within health care is that no one ever asks workers about perceived risks. Hospital policies or guidelines are usually created without significant input from frontline staff. Not only does this cripple an institution's ability to accurately identify issues that are putting patients at risk, but it also leads staff to believe the institution doesn't care about patient safety. When staff reach this unfortunate conclusion, they either accept risk or ignore it, either way, patients continue to be harmed. However, by asking clinicians to identify problems and then supporting their efforts, staff are more likely to embrace problems and try to fix them.

The WICU turned out to be a perfect environment to develop the CUSP model. At the time, it was a new facility that had a large majority of young, relatively inexperienced nurses. This meant that we had far less cultural conditioning to overcome there. The unit had no history; it had no existing culture. It was a blank canvas upon which we could create the culture we believed would foster the best care. Rhonda Wyskiel, who joined the WICU when it first opened, remembers the hunger for change and experimentation that existed then and still exists today.

"We were a staff of nurses fresh out of nursing school working in a new facility. We had the freedom to create whatever systems we wanted. We were eager to cooperate because we witnessed firsthand how change and innovation had improved our work environment," says Rhonda.

Just like TRIP, CUSP starts with the building of a CUSP team. This team oversees the entire process and guides the implementation and management of the program. It's also the driving force in sustaining the program. Each team includes, at minimum, a physician, a nurse, and a senior executive, with associated staff, like pharmacists and respiratory therapists, encouraged to participate. We ask team members to be willing to dedicate four to eight hours per week to the project. New members are encouraged to join at any time.

We ask that the executive be at the vice president level or higher, be available to join the team when it does rounds with patients for one hour per month, and be approachable and comfortable talking about tricky or sensitive topics. In the WICU, hospital president Ron Peterson became our executive team member.

Joining forces with top executives is a powerful tool for change. It bridges the often tense and disconnected gap between top brass and the foot soldiers. It builds morale on the unit because it clearly underlines the fact that the institution actually cares. Executives uniquely hold the power to allocate resources, navigate politics, and increase awareness of issues across the entire hospital landscape.

The senior leaders who serve as CUSP executives often tell me they love this opportunity because it puts them in contact with the real work of a hospital—caring for patients. It's easy for executives to feel cut off and distant from what is happening on the ground level. These executives rarely have any patient care responsibilities; many have no medical education and don't fully understand the finer details of the day-to-day science behind much of what happens on the unit. As such, they can feel out of place visiting a unit. Some of this is due to this unfamiliarity but it is also due to the age-old tension between management and workers, between suits and scrubs. Clinicians often feel that executives only show up on a unit when there's a problem, never as a member of the team to help staff do their jobs. Since we have implemented CUSP, this has changed. The staff has seen how senior executives have embraced problems and facilitated solutions. Similarly, a lot of senior executives tell me their hour on the unit is the appointment they most look forward to each month. I have literally had executives stop me in the halls just to tell me—proudly—that the rates of infection in their unit are still low.

Before launching CUSP in a specific unit we need to get a sense of the existing culture—a baseline, if you will, that we can use to judge improvement. It's not as easy as it sounds. With TRIP, we could measure whether staff did the checklist and we could measure the results of that effort. Culture is a mushy thing to try to gauge. So we turned, once again, to an industry we have turned to a lot in our work: aviation. The airline industry developed a simple survey, the flight management attitudes questionnaire, that effectively rates how well pilots and copilots communicate and work together in the cockpit. Using their survey as a model, a psychologist who worked with our team, Bryan Sexton, developed a similar questionnaire to better learn how staff working on the unit communicate and work together as a team. The survey is called the safety attitudes questionnaire (SAQ). Bryan, through the SAQ, turned this ambiguous concept of culture into something we can measure and thus discuss and improve.

Before administering the survey, we make sure frontline providers understand the purpose of the questionnaire. We make it clear that we want to know what people think of the unit, whether they believe there is good teamwork, if they feel appreciated at work, whether they are able to speak up when they have concerns, if managers address their concerns, and whether they have all that they need to do their jobs effectively. Most importantly, we make sure they understand that the purpose of the exercise is to try to make things better.

Once the survey is completed, we present the results to the unit staff and put together a package for the senior executive. We include detailed information about the CUSP program, results from the SAQ, and pertinent information about the unit that the senior executive may not know (for example, number of beds, staff turnover rate, incident reports, and sentinel events). If we have less than 60 percent compliance with the SAQ, we stop there and send the department chair and medical school dean an e-mail. (This puts a little pressure on staff to participate.) Once we get an acceptable percentage of responses, we are ready to implement CUSP.

With our SAQ scores in hand, we start the "science of safety" training. We recognize that to improve safety, all staff need to understand the "science" that underlies creating safe health care. Most doctors and nurses have no idea how they are harming patients or how to prevent it. If you ask someone whether or not they think they are smart and good at their job, the majority will say yes. We all like to think we are doing our best; we are naturally overconfident. Most of the doctors and nurse I know work very hard and take their work very seriously. Yet, like all humans, we make mistakes, forget things, and sometimes let personality issues prevent us from doing our best work. The health care industry has a strange culture that drives people to believe they are perfect, invincible machines that can work long hours with little sleep and do everything perfectly. It's not until you develop systems designed to root out errors, like CUSP, that the rose-colored glasses fall to the floor. People finally admit to themselves that everybody makes mistakes and if we don't prevent or catch those mistakes, patients will be harmed. Indeed, until they admit this, we have little hope of improving patient safety.

In the science of safety training, we share stories of real patient harm, like the Josie King tragedy. We educate staff about CUSP and what we hope to accomplish. We show them how broken systems and bad culture are the problem, not individuals. We help them learn to "see" broken systems and better understand the basic principles of designing safe systems. We teach them strategies for effective teamwork and communication and help them understand that teams make wise decisions with diverse and independent input. We make it clear that no one from our team is going to dictate which problems should be fixed—or how these issues should be repaired.

Instead members of the unit are going to decide what's broken and how to fix it. We make sure they understand that patient safety can never be fully realized without strong teamwork, communication, and the knowledge and experience each one of them possesses. We further explain that the main purpose of CUSP is to make sure voices are heard, change is made, and patients are safer and each member of the unit is personally accountable for the success of the program. CUSP will provide them with the tools and resources to improve safety, yet they will have to do the work.

Next we set out to identify problems on the unit, what we call defects. We use the word "defects" because the word "errors" is laden with shame and guilt. People make errors—systems have defects. We define defects as anything clinical or operational that you do not want to have happen again. And there are lots of defects—on an average unit, there may be twenty defects a day. For example, a patient has a life-threatening infection and the unit does not have an antibiotic the patient needs—it is supposed to be stocked but it is not there. This forces a nurse to order the antibiotic from the pharmacy, wait a number of hours for the prescription to be filled, and then leave the floor for a half hour to pick it up. This "defect" drastically increases the patient's risk of dying. And yet, it likely happens thousands of times a day in America's hospitals. In fact Sean Berenholtz and I did a study of a sample of hospitals and found that this defect was not only common, but it took, on average, between eight and twenty-four hours to get antibiotics to patients with infections.

When defects like this occur, well-intentioned clinicians work hard to "recover" and make sure the patient is not harmed, but they often do not learn to eliminate or reduce the risks defects pose to future patients. Frontline providers are the eyes and ears of patient safety; they have the expertise and knowledge to see these problems and they are positioned to really effect change. But if there is not a system in place to train them and support them in finding ways to learn from defects, patients continue to be harmed.

Unlike with TRIP, with CUSP we are not looking only for large-scale problems such as bloodstream infections or ventilator-associated pneumonias. In this case a defect could be that the unit doesn't have an operational fax machine and clinicians have to routinely leave patients unattended to go to another floor to fax important documents; or it may be that the unit has a lot of false monitor alarms, leading to confusion and potential patient harm. Even something as mundane as a broken floor tile is a defect if a clinician thinks it might somehow directly or indirectly harm a patient.

Since the overarching goal in CUSP is to improve culture and learn from mistakes, the point here is not only to fix system problems, but also to fix teamwork problems by improving communication and cooperation. The idea is to create a culture of positivity and hope. And hope is often what is missing from burned-out clinicians. If a clinician identifies a problem, speaks up and is heard, and the problem is fixed, that individual feels a part of the win. This not only improves patient safety, it brings joy to the staff and pride to the unit.

When a researcher does not engage members of staff they often don't understand the purpose or benefit of the study. In fact some conclude that the primary goal of the study is to advance the researcher's career. As such, some studies don't get the support they need to be successful. Rhonda knows this very well. "We've had doctors come into our unit and tell us we have to change the way we do things but not explain why. It just adds work to our day and we are already busy so it usually doesn't get a lot of support from staff. Not only that but when they are done they get all the credit and don't even thank us for adding a couple hours a day to our workload."

You do that enough times and cooperation and enthusiasm for new ideas drops to zero. It's important to remember clinicians' first responsibility is to save lives and heal patients; they have their hands full just keeping up with that responsibility. If you want them to take time out of the day to effect change, the staff should be involved to the level where they have ownership, and it should be clear that there is a measurable benefit for the patient.

A little recognition doesn't hurt, either; if people are going to put energy into a project, they deserve credit. Many of the nurses, physicians, and assorted staff who have participated in this work have also been listed as authors on published papers that resulted from our studies. After all, it is their work. Culture is not changed from the top down; it is changed from the inside out. We need everyone on board and everyone working together, equally. Once this is achieved, there's no end to what success you can achieve.

To help clinicians identify problems, we created a basic survey that asked: "How could the next patient be harmed? And what do you think can be done to minimize patient harm or prevent the safety hazard from happening?"

These questions seem simple enough, but hospital culture makes it hard for clinicians to admit they might be harming patients. According to WICU nurse manager Donna Prow, "The nurses on my staff were very uncomfortable with the survey at first. I guess it is because, just like doctors, my nurses didn't believe they, too, could be wrong and could make mistakes. They never thought that they could be doing harm to patients. Of course, once we started looking into improving patient safety, we realized we were making mistakes all the time. What we didn't realize before was that we could and were potentially harming patients."

There is no question hospital errors, no matter what the source, manifest themselves on the front line where medicine meets patient. And the people who best understand what contributes to these errors and how to fix them are these frontline clinicians. Management can help institute the change, provide the needed resources, connect to other units when needed, and help put weight behind the change. But in order to find out where we need to place that pressure, we have to tap into the people who are in direct contact with the patient—the nurses and the doctors. It's not about assessing blame, it's about gathering the tremendous knowledge that frontline providers possess regarding patient risk—knowledge that is all too often overlooked or ignored.

Once the surveys are completed, the CUSP team reviews all the defects and selects a manageable number of problems that have the greatest chance of harming the patient, the highest severity of harm, and the highest frequency of occurrence. The three problems we identified in the WICU were:

1. Safely moving patients to other parts of the hospital (patient transport)
2. Keeping track of prescribed medications (medication reconciliation)
3. Establishing clear communication of the physician's orders (daily goals)

With this list of problems in hand, we held the first of our monthly meetings with our senior executive, shared with him all that we had learned, and began working on solutions. We tried to

meet in the open on the floor—usually as doctors and nurses were
visiting patients and going about their work. We kept these meetings open to anyone on the unit who wanted to attend.

Patient transport was especially difficult in the WICU. This
unit was in a new part of the hospital complex and so it was isolated
from many of the basic services, like CT scans and MRIs. When a
patient needed one of these services, we usually sent a relatively new
nurse and a first-year resident to transport them. The patient had to
be placed on a stretcher, taken down the elevator, wheeled through
a basement hallway the length of several football fields, taken to
the CT scan or other test site, and then wheeled back. This took
substantial time (often several hours) and was risky. We chose two
of the newest members of our staff (a nurse and a resident) because
inexperienced people would be least missed on the unit. Unfortunately it also meant that if something went wrong, these relatively
inexperienced clinicians would be the least likely members of the
team to be able to handle the problem. And as happens with sick
patients, things did go wrong.

Once we had to get an emergency CT scan of a surgical patient on our unit who had lost consciousness. The CT scan machine
is about twenty minutes away, in the basement of one of the other
buildings in the hospital. The patient was on a ventilator and since
we did not have a portable ventilator, we had to manually keep him
breathing using what we call an ambulatory bag, or Ambu bag. Essentially this is a bag that a nurse or doctor squeezes by hand to
force air into the patient's lungs. The problem with this method is
that if it's not done correctly, there is a huge risk of either not delivering enough oxygen to the patient's lungs or hyperventilating the
patient.

When the patient arrived for his CT, there was another scan

in progress and he had to wait for the machine to become available. As they waited, the resident and nurse realized the patient's blood pressure had dropped significantly during transport; before they had time to react, the patient suffered a cardiac arrest. This inexperienced crew had to administer emergency CPR and rush the patient back to the ICU. Luckily the patient survived without harm. However, if a professional transport team had been on board, they would have likely noticed the drop in blood pressure long before the patient had a cardiac arrest. Furthermore it was discovered that the drop in blood pressure was due to a buildup of pressure in the patient's lungs—this acts like a vise around the heart, preventing it from filling with blood. This was probably the result of being hyperventilated on the Ambu bag. The patient was likely given a breath before he had fully exhaled the previous breath, allowing pressure to build up to dangerous levels, and essentially every breath after that was another turn of the vise. Professional transport teams have mobile ventilators that deliver the appropriate amount of oxygen and prevent this kind of thing from happening.

When Ron Peterson heard about our patient transport problem, he couldn't believe an inexperienced nurse and a young resident were routinely charged with pushing very sick patients all over the hospital—often with disastrous consequences. Knowing how busy and short staffed we are, he was equally troubled to learn that these staff members were often missing from the unit for as long as two hours. Sufficiently moved, he did something only a senior executive could do.

At that time Hopkins had started using special transport teams, called "the purple people" because they wore purple uniforms. These teams were made up of nurses who were specifically trained for this kind of work and had the proper equipment to handle almost all emergencies. They were being used by the SICU but had not been assigned to the WICU because originally it was thought the WICU would handle a large population of nonacute patients. Nonacute patients are much healthier and generally are not at great risk during transport. As it turned out, most of our WICU patients were acute and therefore at risk. However, we couldn't just pick up the phone and request purple people. These teams cost money and had to be authorized and cleared by the administration. So Ron Peterson worked with the team to develop a protocol to assess when purple teams were needed (high risk) and when ICU staff could handle the transport (low risk), and he exercised his power to authorize their use.

It was a perfect CUSP team effort. We collectively identified the problem and, thanks to the vision and muscle of our CUSP executive, found a viable solution. The result: the WICU is no longer putting patients at risk during transport.

Medication reconciliation was also a big issue in the WICU, as it was across the hospital. Using the staff survey we showed how more than 75 percent of staff listed medication error as one of the top three ways a patient would be harmed. These errors can easily lead to complications and even death. Studies have shown that one out of five hospital-related injuries are related to errors in drug prescriptions—and half of these errors are tied to medication reconciliation.

We had a patient who was taking medicine, a beta-blocker, to control his heart rate. But when he was transferred to a regular hospital floor, someone forgot to notate that medication. As a result, his heart developed a bad rhythm and he had to be rushed back to our unit, where he spent an additional forty-eight hours. Not only could this man have easily died, but it also added great expense to his care—both for the hospital and the patient.

We had already made a stab at this problem. A couple of years earlier I had invited one of our nurses, Mandy Schwartz, to attend a patient safety conference held by the Institute for Healthcare Improvement (IHI). IHI is one of the early pioneers for patient safety and quality improvement, and much of my early work in patient safety was inspired by its leadership, especially the visionary and charismatic Don Berwick and the chief innovator Tom Nolan. Don engaged health care workers on the need to improve quality of care and Tom was brilliant at designing systems to be safe. I learned much from both of them.

At that conference we heard of a tool IHI had designed to handle the problem of medication reconciliation, so we brought it back to the unit. Though the idea was good, when we presented it to our staff they didn't feel the measurement component was strong enough to tell us whether the tool actually worked. The tool also did not address culture on the unit and predictably, it failed.

This time around, our new CUSP tool had both a strong measurement component that satisfied our nurses and doctors and also addressed culture. The first culture barrier we encountered was that nurses were already very busy and medication reconciliation just added more to their plate. Worse yet, doctors were traditionally supposed to make sure medication orders were correct; the nurses didn't want to have to do what they saw as a "doctor's job" in addition to their own. Turf battles ensued, with doctors and nurses arguing whose job this work was. What was lost in the debate was the patient.

To end these turf battles and get the focus back on the patient, we recounted the story about our patient who had been returned to the unit with an irregular heartbeat because of a medication error. Everyone remembered this story because they had lived it; they saw it with their own eyes. More than anything else, that story helped clinicians really own the problem. It also took the focus away from the battle of doctors versus nurses and put it where it belonged, on patient care.

Once we got our priorities sorted out, we brainstormed the problem and created a form to use for medicine reconciliation. On it we list all the medication the patient was taking before arriving in the unit, what she is taking while in the unit, and what she should take once she leaves the unit. That form never leaves the patient's bedside. It is created and reviewed among caregivers at the time the patient arrives on the unit, numerous times during her stay, and when the patient is scheduled for dismissal from the ICU. If a nurse finds a mistake when reviewing the form, he talks to the physician. If the physician changes the patient's orders as a result of that discussion, we record it as an error. Our goal is to be error free.

As simple as this sounds, nothing like this existed on the unit or in health care before. The Joint Commission now requires all hospitals have some system in place to reconcile medications. However there is no standardization of these systems and not all are effective, which means patients are likely still being harmed.

As important as it was to address and fix our problems with patient transport and medication reconciliation, far and above the biggest success story that came out of using CUSP in the WICU was the birth of our daily goals form. Communication of the care team's daily goals was a big problem in the WICU (as it was in almost every unit in any hospital anywhere). Members of the care team, especially nurses, were often not clear on the physicians' treatment plan or goals for the patient. When ambiguity exists on this level, confused nurses must continuously ask physicians questions—thus raising tensions in the unit, slowing the workflow, and putting patients in danger.

To understand the magnitude of this problem, I must first explain how care is delivered in a Hopkins ICU. An attending physician, like me, is in charge. Every day we walk around the unit with the nurses, the nurse practitioners, the fellows (doctors training to be an attending), the residents (doctors training to be an attending or fellow), and medical students (training to be a resident). The chief resident or nurse practitioner introduces the patient and recommends a care plan and the attending summarizes and defines the final plan for each patient. Traditionally these are given verbally and the chief resident writes them down.

Since I'm an attending physician in the WICU, when I heard that my rounds were not effective, it got my attention. I was concerned first because of the risk to the patient, but second because this problem was clearly the result of a bad system I was likely helping to perpetuate. Eager to further sound out this problem I decided to try a little test. (It was so successful that I now do this all the time.) I asked one of the nurses to watch while we gave rounds and tell us what she observed. She had participated in the science of safety training so she knew what to look for—a culture or systems issue that might lead to patient harm. When we were done with rounds, I asked her to tell us if she had seen anything. I thought I had done a good job so I wasn't expecting her to tell me much. To my surprise she had a look of bewilderment and disbelief on her face.

She replied, "Didn't anyone else see it? The nurse in charge of one of the patients was talking about his care when a resident came in and stood directly between her and Dr. Pronovost. She stopped talking after that, and nobody even noticed."

I turned to the nurse in question and asked her, "Is this true?"

She responded, "Yes."

"How did that make you feel?" I asked.

"I was embarrassed and humiliated," the nurse admitted. "I felt like what I had to say didn't matter."

I was shocked that I hadn't noticed, and neither had the residents or the other nurses. We all apologized and honestly told the nurse that we didn't mean to interrupt her or ignore her, but it was clear this kind of thing happens all the time and the nurses have just grown to expect it. Curious, I asked the nurse what it was she was going to say when she was cut off.

She said, "The patient's blood platelet count is very low."

These blood results had only just come in and she was the only one who knew about it. If I had missed this, I would have stopped the blood thinner, which could have harmed this patient. It only made me wonder how many thousands of times vital information falls through cracks because of simple oversights like this.

This type of problem starts in medical school and nursing school, where doctors aren't trained to listen to nurses and nurses aren't trained to ask questions or believe they play an important role in the patient's care. Rhonda calls this kind of blind obedience being a "task mongrel."

"Nurses are taught that if a doctor writes an order, you do it. I tell my nurses, don't ever be a task mongrel. Never carry out an order without knowing why you are doing it. Never give a patient anything without knowing why you are giving it," she says.

I must admit my ego was bruised when I learned that communication between members of the care team was so obviously flawed. But I was willing to accept that this needed to change. I knew the first step was to get a clear idea of exactly how bad the problem was. So we developed a simple survey. After spending fifteen minutes discussing a patient on our round, we asked the nurses and residents whether they could tell us the goals of care for that patient that day and what needed to happen for the patient to leave the ICU. Much to my shock, only 6 percent of residents and 5 percent of nurses felt they could give us a clear answer. It was obvious we had a big problem.

So we looked at our methods to see if we could improve them. The standard model for making rounds is the attending physician announces the patient's treatment while the head resident scribbles it down. The hope is that the resident gets it down correctly and that everyone else hears it as well. Most of the time the patient's nurse is not present on rounds and does not even hear the plan.

We changed the model to require that the patient's nurse be present during rounds and that rounds not start without him or her. We developed a clear, easy-to-read care plan form that the resident fills out at the end of rounds and the nurse then reads back—confirming there are no communication errors. The system is not without flaws, but it is substantially better than our prior system. The resident and attending still brainstorm about diagnosis and treatment. Yet at the end we create a concrete, unambiguous plan and ensure all members of the team are aware and agree with it. And most importantly, everyone provides input to both the brainstorming discussion and the plan.

This new system ensures that we don't have conflicting orders— such as a cardiologist wanting a patient to have less fluids to relieve heart failure and a nephrologist requesting more fluids to increase blood flow to the kidneys. With the daily goals sheet, if there were such a conflict, questions would be asked and it would be resolved during rounds while everyone was present. In the past, the care plan would not be clear, so nurses would be confused and would inevitably page a number of doctors, wasting time and potentially placing a patient at risk.

At first, some attending physicians refused to use the daily goals sheet, claiming they did not need it. But luckily it started to catch on. I was the first to use it. Nurses and residents embraced it next and soon believed in it so strongly they demanded other physicians use it. Eventually, everyone found it useful.

Like many new initiatives, in the beginning using the daily goals form seemed like it took more time. But once confusion in the care plan and incidents of paging decreased, doctors and nurses alike realized they were actually saving time using the daily goals sheet and the patient was getting better care. You cannot force culture change. A tool, such as the daily goals form, must have self-evident value; staff should understand why it is being used and sense (or better measure) that care is better. Everyone needs to understand the tool and feel free to revise it if they think it can be improved. The daily goals form is now being used in thousands of ICUs around the world, and it is likely saving lives and money.

After implementing all of our CUSP solutions, we measured performance. We measured whether the culture improved and we measured whether the new interventions helped fix the problems we had identified. The results were staggering:

1. Our safety culture scores (on the survey) went up by 50 percent.
2. The length of stay for our patients dropped by half, to just over one day—unprecedented for an ICU that cares for sick surgical patients.
3. Medication errors dropped from 94 percent to almost zero.
4. Nursing turnover decreased from 9 percent to 2 percent.

At the time this was likely the most rigorous culture measurement performed at a hospital. Our response rate across the ICU was over 70 percent. But easily the most important result of this work was the effect it had on the unit. It wasn't just that we improved a couple of targeted problems; the entire mood of the unit was enhanced. Everyone felt energized and privileged to be working in the WICU. Their voices were heard and change really happened. Each member of the team played a role and had a right to take credit for our successes.

"We were part of the change. It wasn't like someone was telling us to do this or do that. We played a role in making those decisions. These were our changes, too. It was actually fun to come to work just to find out in what new ways we could make our unit safer for patients," says Rhonda.

Having solid, measured results is a key element to all this work. For one, if you don't have reliable numbers, the medical community won't believe that what you did actually works. But results have another important effect on a project. Positive results further inspire the people who do the work. In this case the doctors and the nurses in the WICU. Everyone likes to win. And there's no way to know whether the team has won or not if you don't measure results.

Furthermore, when winning means that patients receive better care, it's a double win for health care workers. Everyone I know in health care wants to deliver the best possible care to patients. This is what gets us out of bed in the morning, what inspires us to pull twelve-, sixteen-, twenty-, or twenty-four-hour workdays. It's why we signed up in the first place. When the team in the WICU had real proof that our efforts actually paid off, it made our spirits soar. It made us eager to strive for even higher plateaus. It's that energy that makes our work continue to expand and prosper. It's what made it possible for us to translate our successes in one small ICU unit at Johns Hopkins to the entire Michigan health care system.

# Chapter 5

W hen I was invited to speak at a health care conference in Michigan I had no idea we would soon be applying our program to that entire state's health care system. In fact that conference got off to a rather bad start.

Michigan was not new to patient safety work. On the contrary, the state was, and still is, on the vanguard of health care reform. There was a strong relationship in the state between the principal employers (the large automakers), the insurers (primarily Blue Cross), and the care providers (the hospitals). The automakers had been trying to reduce health care costs for over a decade and this had helped motivate both the insurers and providers to improve quality and reduce costs.

I was intimately aware of this community. Early in my patient safety career, I published my Ph.D. thesis in the *Journal of the American Medical Association* (*JAMA*) demonstrating that surgical patients having aortic surgery had a 39 percent lower mortality rate and a 29 percent shorter length of stay when treated in the ICU by an intensivist and surgeon team rather than by a surgeon alone. The Leapfrog Group, a national consortium of over one hundred Fortune 500 companies that sought to improve health care, chose this idea as one of three programs it believed would have the greatest impact on improving quality and lowering health care costs for its member companies. At the time, only 5 to 10 percent of patients in the ICU were cared for by intensivists. Arnie Milstein, the medical director of the Leapfrog Group, asked me if I would come to General Motors' headquarters to talk about my *JAMA* study. What he didn't tell me was that he had also invited the CEOs and chief medical officers from the fourteen largest health care insurers in the country.

Before I was introduced, the executive director of GM said that when they have a death on the shop floor from injury, they close the shop, investigate, and fix what was wrong, and as a result they have a good safety record. Yet he was shocked to learn that GM employees, retirees, and dependents died every day because ICUs lacked intensivists and nothing was being done about it.

He closed by stating, "We are not going to tolerate this anymore, and Dr. Pronovost will tell you why."

It had been inspiring to see industry and insurers taking such an interest in patient safety. And, given the reputation the state had for this work, I was sure I would have a similar experience this time around. The MHA Insurance Company—a large company that insured many physicians in the state—had organized the conference and had invited patient safety experts from all over the country. I was eager to meet and share ideas with these experts, as well as representatives from many of the hospitals in the state.

The talk was scheduled for early Monday, February 10, the day after my daughter's third birthday. The insurance company had me booked on a six-hour connecting flight the previous evening so I could have dinner with some of the conference organizers. I was not happy about these arrangements because I was going to miss my daughter's party. When I arrived at the airport, that unhappiness turned to anger and frustration when I realized there were a handful of direct flights that would have gotten me to Detroit in an hour, enabling me to make both the dinner and my daughter's party. I called the travel agency and they told me the insurance company had instructed them to book me on the cheapest flight. For a savings of twenty dollars the organizers of the conference had forced me to miss my daughter's birthday party and waste five hours of my time.

I almost turned around and went home. However, I knew there were a lot of people in Michigan waiting to learn about our work. I had to remind myself that this trip was about making hospitals safer, not about my ego. So I got on the plane. To make matters worse, my flight was delayed two hours in Chicago and didn't get into Detroit until midnight—too late for the dinner. I dragged my tired body through the cold and empty airport searching for a place to eat (I hadn't eaten since breakfast). But every food concession I passed was closed for the night. When I eventually checked in to the hotel, room service had also shut down. My dinner consisted of a package of stale peanut M&Ms I scavenged from my hotel room's minibar.

When I walked into the conference center the next morning, I was approached by an energetic woman who quickly introduced herself as Chris Goeschel. Chris was the director of a not-for-profit organization, the Keystone Center for Patient Safety, whose sole purpose was to address quality and safety issues within the state. The Keystone Center was part of the Michigan Hospital Association (MHA), which represented over a hundred hospitals, ranging from small community hospitals to large academic centers similar to Hopkins. MHA and MHA Insurance Company were loosely connected through some shared board members.

Chris had read a lot of the published literature on our research, especially about our CUSP and TRIP work. And (although I didn't know it at the time) she had been talking to MHA about implementing our program in the entire state of Michigan.

I was still steaming about the flight to Detroit, so as soon as she finished introducing herself, I launched into her: "I have to be honest, I'm a little upset. Someone in your organization booked me on what turned out to be a seven-hour flight from Baltimore to save twenty dollars, when I could have easily gotten here in one hour. Because of this, you wasted my time and I missed my daughter's party. Frankly, I would never think of putting someone who I invite to talk on a connecting flight when a direct one is available."

She didn't even flinch. She just stood there smiling and took my assaults graciously. When I was done, she said, "Dr. Pronovost, please accept my deepest apologies for what has obviously been a terrible mistake. I will do my best to look into this issue for you. My organization didn't make the arrangements; they were handled by the insurance company that paid for the flight."

She then excused herself, only to return fifteen minutes later.

"Dr. Pronovost, we have you booked on a direct, first-class flight that leaves right after your talk; a car service will be waiting to drive you to the airport. Once again, please accept our apologies."

I was still angry, but her graciousness had put me on the road to recovery.

The talk went exceeding well. I shared our successes at Hopkins and told the audience I was positive these results could easily be accomplished at other hospitals. The conference reenergized me, as did Chris's efforts to assuage my anger. As I was leaving, she approached me again.

"Dr. Pronovost, I speak for everyone when I say we are all very impressed. I have been following your work closely and I want to ask you if you would be interested in implementing your program across the entire state of Michigan. I have spoken with the ICU directors at many of our hospitals and they are eager to improve safety and want to use your program. They respect your work because they believe it is based in a scientific approach that produces valid data with real results. Just as you did at Hopkins, we need to improve the quality of ICU care here and we think your program could provide us with the tools we need to accomplish that goal."

If Chris had asked me that question only a couple of hours earlier I would have given her an absolute no. But her positive energy, her persistence, her kindness, her passion about safety, and her genuine nature won me over. I didn't say yes. But I did tell her I would think about it. Even if they hadn't screwed up my flight, I would have had mixed feelings. On one hand, I was ecstatic about the potential to improve care in a whole state. On the other hand, I was terrified; nobody had done this before.

This bizarre start to my relationship with Michigan and Chris is just one example of how good fortune propelled this work forward against some pretty serious odds. It's as if there is an angel watching over us ready to catch us any time we are about to become discouraged or stumble. A study I read about showed that people's moods improved 70 percent when they ate chocolate that had received positive prayers by monks versus similar chocolate that had not received these prayers. The researchers hypothesize that we are all connected through energy, and that good intentions—such as the monks' prayers—are palpable and influential. Perhaps our guardian angel is good intentions. The health care workers at Hopkins and those I met in Michigan all seemed to have good intentions. All of them had put in a lot of hours on the front line and seemed to have a sincere desire to find ways to improve care. Similarly, Chris worked as a nurse for many years before she became an administrator. She, like many others, spent many hours dealing with bad culture and broken systems. People like Chris chose health care as a career because they wanted to help patients.

I sensed an immediate connection with this dynamic woman. First, she was one of the few people who had the energy to keep up with my pace. Second, she was deeply committed to the work. For her, this was not about publishing papers or getting visibility; it was about reducing preventable harm. She felt the same moral obligation to do the work that I did. At the conference, Chris inspired me to think big. She has continued to do that ever since. If it weren't for Chris's tenacity and vision, the project in Michigan would have never happened. But it did.

Six months after that awkward discussion at the MHA conference, we received a two-year grant from the Agency for Healthcare Research and Quality to reduce bloodstream infections in the ICUs across Michigan using the CUSP and TRIP models. Of course, it wasn't easy getting there. In order to win the grant we had put together a two-hundred-page competitive proposal in record time. The seed was planted, the synergy had begun, and all that was left was a lot of hard work. Between Chris and me, our schedules didn't permit another face-to-face meeting, so we put that proposal together with thousands of e-mails and frequent calls. We learned about the grant in June and our deadline for the grant proposal was early July. As a result, Chris and I worked round the clock through the July Fourth weekend struggling to meet the deadline. It came right down to the wire. Between grilling burgers and jumping in the pool with my kids, I was writing the grant and on the phone with Chris.

But it wasn't just us two who were energized. The entire state was responding. We got fifty ICU units to sign up in six months, and another forty-nine signed up by the time we launched the project in October. And even more joined after that. Momentum was building daily; the pressure was on. The entire state of Michigan was counting on us.

As my universe was expanding I needed help, so we created the Johns Hopkins Quality and Safety Research Group (QSRG) and I became its director. The staff included a highly trained team of physicians, nurses, health service researchers, science writers, organizational psychologists, and hospital infection control physicians, as well as several faculty in the School of Public Health. For the Michigan project, QSRG joined forces with Chris and her staff from MHA's Keystone Center. We provided the technical knowledge and experience with the program and MHA managed the implementation of the program at each of the hospitals in the state.

We ran the Michigan program as a collaborative. In this method, groups are brought together to solve problems. We planned on having a series of conference calls and biannual group meetings with the various ICU teams in the state to disseminate information, build teamwork, and share knowledge. For a project of this magnitude, running a collaborative program was really the only option. While this method was very popular with safety programs, collecting accurate data has traditionally been a problem. This concerned us since collecting good data is a key component of our work. At the end of the day, patients and providers want and deserve to know whether the effort actually improved safety.

Another obstacle was deciding how to assemble all the work we had done at Hopkins into a single program that we could export to Michigan. At Hopkins we used TRIP to eliminate bloodstream infections and CUSP to build teamwork, and we believed teams needed to do both to be successful. Yet, we never ran them together as we planned to do in Michigan. It all made sense in my head but we needed to come up with a new strategy if we were going to tackle hospitals across Michigan.

Whatever strategy we used, it would have to be flexible. At Hopkins we had the luxury of working in a homogeneous environment that we knew and understood well, whereas in Michigan, we would be dealing with large academic medical centers and small community hospitals—each with unique strengths and weaknesses. Academic hospitals are bigger organizationally and therefore much more complex. We know from our research that the bigger the hospital, the more layers of culture you have and the harder it is to change that culture. However, academic centers often have critical care doctors committed solely to the ICU, making it easier to arrange group rounds, standardize care and promote teamwork. On the flip side, small community facilities often depend on doctors who have private practices and are not tied directly to the hospital, which can complicate teamwork and quality improvement efforts. Yet since most community hospitals are small, the culture is limited to a manageable number of players, making easier to evoke change.

With these challenges in mind we decided to apply the measurement and the checklist aspects of our TRIP model in a central fashion and the unit-based culture work of our CUSP model locally. The logic behind this was that checklist and measurement were fairly straightforward and required little interpretation or adaptation. More to the point, it was essential that everyone knew the evidence supporting the items on the checklist and that measurement was uniform across the state. Conversely, culture issues and barriers, as we know, vary greatly across health care organizations. Since we would be working with large teaching hospitals, small community hospitals, and some in between, there would be a lot of variation between staff and units; one set of universal rules just wouldn't work for this part of the program. Finding this delicate balance between central and local efforts was key to our success.

Our program would begin with a couple of introductory conference calls. The purpose of these calls was to give a general outline of the program—the science of safety, items on the checklist, TRIP and CUSP theory, and instructions on how to collect data. We would talk about what these programs had accomplished at Johns Hopkins and what we hoped to accomplish in Michigan. We wanted Michigan to understand that this was hard work and we all had much to learn. We wanted to be sure that participants recognize that Johns Hopkins had not solved all its safety problems and we would be struggling along with them trying to find our collective way.

The idea of rolling out this program across an entire state at both small and large hospitals was nerve-racking enough. But to get on the phone with hundreds of people, all waiting to hear the first words about how we would pull off this historic project, added a whole extra level of stress. This was the first time most of these people had heard of us or had a chance to learn anything substantive about our program. Considering how much resistance my team had experienced at Hopkins, we knew that we would also have a lot of skeptics in Michigan. First impressions are everything and we knew this first call could make or break us. In other words, this call had to be really good.

I started by introducing myself. "Hello, my name is Peter Pronovost. Thank you for . . ." But before I could get out another word, a hiss of deafening, ear-piercing static filled the phone line and made it impossible to speak or hear. When it went away I assumed it was just a glitch so I started again, and the same thing happened. At first

I thought it was human error so I started getting frustrated. Chris and I were not in the same room; she was in Michigan and I was in Baltimore. We had only been working together for a short time, I did not know her competencies, and we were just beginning to trust each other.

I called out to Chris, who was somewhere in Michigan in this sea of callers: "Chris, can you fix this problem?"

Chris replied, "We are working on it; we called the operator."

But when the problem persisted, I demanded, "Chris, could you please ask the operator to get us a new line? We need to figure out what is going on."

"Peter, I am working on it."

Chris had her staff called the phone company, technical experts, the conference call company—anyone they could think of that might be able to help. Meanwhile we had hundreds of people waiting, listening. To make things even worse, we didn't set up the call correctly so that when anyone went on hold, the entire group could hear "hold" music, which only added to the confusion.

It appeared as though our first attempt at a conference call was turning into a disaster. Since our program asked a lot from these teams, we needed to earn their trust and cooperation. Yet, because of technical difficulties, we sounded like a bunch of amateurs. Eventually, Chris found out what was going on and got back on the line.

She said, "Peter, we found out what the problem is and it is beyond our control. The entire country is experiencing the same thing—solar flares."

When I heard this I spontaneously burst out laughing. It was a critical moment; the other people on the line could have interpreted my response unfavorably, but by some stroke of luck my laughter was infectious. What I hadn't realized was that everyone on the call was as nervous as I was. As bad as the solar flares and hold music had been, the laughter disarmed a lot of clinicians who were most likely coming into this with suspicions and doubts. Instead of being intimidated by me, these doctors and nurses realized I was just as human as they were, just as prone to making mistakes. The fact that we didn't have everything figured out was precisely the point. It became a catalyst for synergy—everyone seemed to realize that we were all struggling to make this happen and that it wouldn't work unless we worked together. As we went forward with the Michigan program, that spirit endured.

Our calls were part religious revival and part science class. Everybody on the call had to become familiar with the technical portions of the program: the science of safety, CUSP, TRIP, and all the research tools associated with better teamwork. Everybody had to know the evidence behind our central line checklists. But we also knew they would quickly get bored with science lectures. We needed to energize and inspire them, to make them believe that they could actually change care and get these infection rates down, that these infections were largely preventable. We wanted them to believe that they could lead their hospital effort and that they were participating in something much bigger than themselves—a statewide effort. We had no doubt they would succeed.

CUSP not only inspired teamwork and improved culture and communication. It also helped influence our critics to get on board with the program. Instead of seeing this work as some random policy imposed on them from some relatively unknown physician from a hospital a thousand miles away, staff at each hospital saw it as their own. They worked on problems specific to their hospital and their unit, and they were free to decide on their own what solutions they would use to fix those problems.

In this regard, what we did at Michigan was essentially a prov-
erb come to life: "Give a man a fish and he'll eat for a day; teach him
to fish and he'll eat for a lifetime." We didn't want to impose just
another new safety initiative, designed to address one problem that
would be ignored and then discarded. We wanted to give hospital
staff in Michigan the tools they needed to address any and all safety
problems they faced today or would face in the future.

What we didn't expect to see was CUSP and TRIP morphing
into one program, which is essentially what it is today. (Now we
would never think of implementing one without the other.) Since
we didn't and really couldn't control the way each hospital used
our system, we soon found that some started CUSP first and then
moved on to TRIP, while others jumped right into TRIP and then
did CUSP later. As the program moved forward the two essentially
blended together. But this is not surprising. They do not live without
each other. And in fact they overlap considerably. Trying to put evidence into practice without changing culture is like Sisyphus trying
to push a rock up a hill. It's labor-intensive and you'll never reach
your goal. On the other hand, improving culture without having a
clear checklist, with the science and measurement to back it up, is
like a "Kumbaya" session. It might raise the spirits but nothing really
is getting done; and at the end of the day, you do not know if you are
really making things any safer.

We had calls once a week for the first few months, just to get
things going, and then monthly. Generally the telephone conversations consisted of twenty minutes of disseminating information,
usually by me or one of the other safety experts on our team, and
the rest of the hour would be interactive. I would ask Chris to
query the groups and find the best examples of what worked and
what was not working and ask these teams to present. In this way

teams began talking to each other, sharing tips about what they did to solve the problems presented by other teams. I took the role as a mediator, facilitating the conversation but mostly listening and learning.

On one of our calls a tiny community hospital in northern Michigan, which had only four beds in its ICU, talked about how it had amazing success standardizing its central line catheter procedures. Conversely, one of the largest hospitals in the state said it was struggling. As we listened, the large, well-known hospital asked this small, obscure community hospital for help with this problem, and got it. These kinds of exchanges were powerful and highly effective, both for improving patient outcomes and ensuring the overall success of the program. Instead of dismissing advice based on the source, the larger institution listened humbly and intently, implemented the techniques, and had amazing results. This was just the kind of community, and access to information, we were trying to create.

But of course the calls were not all smooth sailing. Just as we had experienced at Hopkins, there was a good bit of resistance. At one point in a call, a frustrated doctor from a large hospital center asked me, "Why are you making us do this? We have already reduced our central line infections. You are wasting my valuable time! We don't need to add just one more program to our already busy schedules, and frankly there is no scientific evidence supporting your methods. I don't know why you even brought me in on this call."

The whole state was listening as this highly respected doctor openly challenged the entire program, as was I. I had experienced this kind of resistance at Hopkins and felt I had a pretty clear idea where it was coming from. This was not about me or my program— it was about him. It was about loss. He felt as if he was losing his authority. My response was, "It sounds like you really did a great job there. Maybe you can speak at the next session and tell everyone how you did it. When you come, please bring your data."

The doctor responded happily, "Sure, I'll bring the data."

"Also, when you go to gather your data," I added, "look at two things. Look at how complete your data is and if you used the standardized definitions of bloodstream infections from the CDC. When you come to present, be sure to share with the whole group what you did, the results you achieved, and how confident you are in your data." There was a silence on the phone and then, a few seconds later, he thanked me for the invitation.

The doctor never presented his data at any of our meetings. Instead, he came up to me, alone, in private, at the next meeting and said, "Thanks. When I looked at our data it was junk; there was about 60 percent missing data and the data we had, who knows how it was collected. I want you to know I am in. I want this to be good science."

I was glad that he had decided to join us. However, this encounter was a classic example of the cultural barriers that keep physicians cut off from engaging in patient safety efforts and from learning from other clinicians. He was comfortable sharing with me alone that he was wrong about the level of care he delivered, that patients were still being harmed from infections at his hospital. But he was not comfortable sharing this publicly. Doctors go into medicine to help rather than harm patients. And they feel a deep sense of shame to think they have failed—a shame they suffer privately. We need to remove this yoke of guilt so they can learn from mistakes and defects in the workplace, and create a culture that not only fixes problems and helps clinicians learn from each other, but catches errors before they harm patients. Until we do this we will never be able to fix these systems—we will constantly be looking at the wrong end of the horse.

A call came to me personally from a small, rural hospital in the Upper Peninsula that only had a two-bed ICU and didn't have intensivists. An emergency care doctor at that hospital really wanted to do our program but he was worried that since it did not have intensivists on staff we would not let his hospital into the program.

"I know you have published on a intensivist-staffed ICU model," he said. "Are you going to kick us out of the program because we do not have intensivists?"

I replied, "Of course not. You have to operate with the resources you have. Since you don't have the money to hire intensivists, just make sure the doctors who take care of patients in the ICU have the following skills: they're present in the ICU; they're knowledgeable about how to treat critically ill patients; they communicate with other staff and family; and they create and use guidelines, protocols, and admission and discharge criteria."

That rural ICU not only joined the program, but decreased its infection rate to nearly zero. In place of intensivists, the hospital trained emergency physicians and hospitalists. A hospitalist is similar to an intensivist, only these doctors generally look after the overall care of patients on the floor instead of the ICU. This is a perfect example of an individual team innovating and adapting to the model based on resources available.

We also had some problems with the way infectious disease practitioners viewed central line infections. Up until now, all bloodstream infections were their turf. They believed they owned the problem, not the doctors and nurses in the ICU. This sense of ownership removed accountability from these ICU clinicians. And experience had taught us that if you don't get ICU clinicians to take responsibility for these infection rates, the rates aren't likely to be reduced. Infection disease practitioners had exceptional knowledge and training regarding these infections. We desperately needed their expertise. But just as we had learned at Hopkins, we needed the ultimate accountability to fall on the ICU physicians who were actually placing central lines in the patients, where the patient met the procedure.

So we made the ICU clinicians accountable and placed the infectious disease experts in a critical yet supportive role. The infectious disease experts could help train and educate, robustly monitor infections, investigate when and why infections occurred, and provide technical support; yet the doctors and nurses who worked in the ICU had to accept responsibility for infections. We felt this was the best way to get the ICU doctors and nurses, and the infectious disease experts, all to participate. Without this kind of collaborative effort—without teamwork, without knowledge sharing—the situation would never get any better.

As I started implementing this plan, I quickly learned, through Chris, that some of the infectious disease people were angry with me and would not support these efforts. This was my fault. I had spent most of my time engaging ICU doctors and nurses, and had neglected doing the same for the infectious disease teams. At Hopkins I worked closely with, and depended on, Dr. Trish Perl and Dr. Sara Cosgrove, who lead our infection control efforts. And I knew I would need to have the same approach in Michigan if I wanted these teams to support our work.

The infectious disease community in Michigan is exceedingly well organized and highly talented. Its members include leaders of both national and international professional societies and advisers to the CDC. I asked Chris if we could arrange a call with Michigan's infectious disease experts and invite the group to our collaborative meeting. I knew the initial call was going to be challenging and I would have to leave my ego checked at the door. When I received blows I would have to stay poised and not react. I had to remember that the goal was to improve safety; and we were aligned on that goal. I also had to try to understand why these doctors were having difficulty with our work. I had to see this problem from their perspective. Only then could I better understand what motivated them and hopefully persuade them to take their place helping to lead the efforts.

The call was difficult. I was outnumbered about twelve to one. At first I just listened; the infectious disease doctors challenged me on technical issues; I listened. They challenged me on turf issues; I listened.

After about thirty minutes, I asked, "Do you think we should infect patients in Michigan?"

A clear "No" followed.

"Do you think we can substantially reduce these infections?" I asked. There was silence. I said, "I do. I have seen the program work. But it will not work without your leadership and technical expertise. If you have concerns with technical details, tell me and we can discuss the issues. I understand I am new at trying to reduce infections and that you have been laboring at this for decades. I do not pretend to be a technical expert. Yet I believe I have an approach to improving safety that works. It is hard work and requires your input. If we succeed here and are able to save lives and money—and I am certain we can—you will have the support you need from your CEOs to do more work. More importantly, you will have accomplished what you have been working to achieve for years: preventing health care–acquired infections."

The ice began to thaw, and by the end of that call, we agreed to collaborate. It was understandable that these highly trained professionals be skeptical. They were scientists; it was their job to question new theories and ideas. I couldn't expect them to participate without effectively presenting the evidence they needed to better understand the program. Now that we had talked, now that they had a better understanding of the science, the infectious disease doctors were on board. Internally I breathed a sigh of relief. Our work would have been impossible without the help of the infectious disease doctors and nurses.

In spite of these pockets of resistance, our calls went very well. People were talking and learning, and enthusiasm was growing. After six or seven of these calls, we were ready for our first face-to-face meeting. I had never met these teams. I was actually quite nervous because I didn't really know what to expect.

The night before our first meeting, I had worked the night shift in the ICU. I finished work at six a.m. and got on a plane to Michigan. Chris and I wanted to keep these meetings loose and flexible. Often we were preparing in the last few hours before we presented—trying to adjust to the latest issues that had surfaced and ideas that had percolated in our calls. In this spirit, I put the finishing touches on my talk during the early morning flight. I e-mailed the files to Chris when my plane touched down and she got them printed and put into binders to hand out after the meeting, which started at eight a.m.

Chris had sent a car to take me to the conference. I was tired and looking a little scruffy. I remember seeing an older gentleman with a sign that read, DR. PRONOVOST.

I went up to him and said, "I think you are looking for me."

The man took one look at me and said, "No, sonny, I am waiting for an important doctor from Johns Hopkins."

"Yes, I know," I said. "That would be me."

The driver looked at me again and said, "No, sonny, you don't understand. I was sent here to pick up a famous Johns Hopkins doctor."

At this point, feeling exhausted, I just started laughing and said, "Sorry to disappoint you, that's me. Let's go."

When I walked into the conference room and stood on stage, it was nothing short of amazing. I was staring out at five hundred doctors and nurses who were hungry to make a difference in the world and looking for how to do it. I was not really sure how we were going to get there. We had hunches, theory, and experience, but no clear plan. This was new. The energy in that room told me the audience just wanted someone to help them believe that they could improve patient care. We have since come to learn that engendering that belief is often 90 percent of the battle. Clinicians, especially nurses, so often feel beaten down, unappreciated, and ineffective. When professionals like these get no voice in improving care, little valid data about performance, and few resources to work with, they may well become apathetic. Yet when clinicians sense that someone believes in them, believes without a doubt that they can improve care, they live up to that belief.

I opened up my presentation, as I always do, with a picture of Josie King.

I promised this little girl's mother that our work will actually make hospitals safer so tragedies like this are less likely to occur. How can we do that? Our goal is to answer that question, not just for Sorrel King, but for the citizens of Michigan, the United States, and the world. To date, no one has been able to answer that question on a large scale. If we are successful we will be the first. Michigan can demonstrate to the world that high-quality care is achievable not just in a select few hospitals, not just in marketing materials, but for all its citizens; and then back it up with credible data. It will require hard work and discipline but with courage, commitment, and clarity we can get the job done. We are going to prove to the citizens of Michigan that we can reduce the risk of infections in the ICU. We will ensure that no matter which hospital Michiganders choose for their care, they will not suffer a bloodstream infection in the ICU. We did it at Hopkins, and we have an obligation to help hospitals and patients everywhere achieve the same goal. It is immoral to withhold information that might help improve the care of a patient. If one hospital manages to get its infection rates down and the hospital across town still has high numbers, the staff of the first hospital should and must reach out to the failing hospital and lend a helping hand. We will not judge our success based on how each hospital performs, but on how the entire state does as whole. I, too, have looked at medicine as a competitive business. My mother always goes to her local hospital because she knows and trusts the people there. As a young doctor at Hopkins I often wished that she would seek out a large academic institution. Since I worked in one, I knew and trusted those institutions more than community hospitals. I believed we delivered a better product. For rare diseases for which little is known, the expertise of multiple specialists is needed. But for much of medicine, for conditions we know how to diagnose and treat with a reasonable degree of accuracy, we should be able to trust that all hospitals everywhere deliver the same level of care. Why should a patient have to fear that a hospital will accidentally cut off the wrong leg or not know about a drug or treatment that will cure his disease? That's nuts. We don't choose airlines based on which ones we think will not crash. Why should health care be different? The way to reach this goal is for all of us to join together. We must learn and share together. Each of you has something to offer, whether you are a community hospital with a two-bed ICU or a large medical center with a fifteen-bed ICU. If you are succeeding, help a neighbor. If we can make this happen here in Michigan, we can make it happen across the country and the world. It's up to us to show everyone else the way.

Every meeting was different, but usually we had a series of speakers from Hopkins, Keystone, and hospitals throughout the state. We showed numerous inspirational clips like films of Roger Bannister, the runner who first broke the four-minute mile, and the 1980 U.S. hockey team that, against all odds, managed to beat the Russian team and win the Olympic gold. Between speeches, I would roam the crowd with a wireless microphone taking questions and hearing stories. As I walked around we energized each other; as we shared stories and experiences it helped ease their self-doubts and mine as well. To be honest, I was not sure we could improve care in a whole state. It had never been done before. And that made me both excited and anxious. But in spite of our collective doubts, there was no turning back. Momentum was building and we all knew we were going to push until we reached our goal of eliminating infections in the state, whatever it took.

In this fashion, many of the meetings were filled with tears of inspiration, laughter, and boundless energy. Despite often showing up sleep deprived from working in the ICU, I always left energized.

Like most efforts in life in which you seek to make the world better, I received much more than I gave. In the end we were all working together trying to find answers to the same question—how can we help make patients safer?

It was crucial that we saw ourselves as one united team. In this spirit Chris printed up T-shirts that listed every single hospital in the program. Similarly, all of our correspondence, every single letter, fax, or handout, was printed on stationery that also listed these hospitals. If a team wanted to let us know they were struggling to collect data, we asked that it be printed on this stationery. We wanted everyone to be constantly reminded that they were part of this team and by failing to work harder they would be letting the whole team down.

As time went on, this sense of family began to have a name, "Ohana." The name came out of the Disney cartoon *Lilo and Stitch*, which my daughter, Emma, loved to watch at the time. In the movie a young Hawaiian girl loses her parents and depends on the care and love of her older sister. At one point a potential husband courts the older sister, and the little girl is fearful the sister will marry and abandon her. The older sister tells the young child that she was protected by *ohana*—a Hawaiian word for "family" that essentially means, "You won't be left behind."

As I watched the movie one night with my daughter, Emma, I made a direct connection between the movie and our work in Michigan. Our work, like this movie, was about family and communities. It was a powerful emotional moment. The next morning, while running, I reflected on what I would say at the Michigan meeting the next day—*ohana* came to mind. The word soon became our slogan for teamwork. At one very emotional session, the teams presented me with a baseball cap that they had made with the word "Ohana" printed on it. Chris also found a soft drink brand named Ohana that we purchased and distributed to the group.

Ohana swept thorough the Michigan health care system like a fresh breeze energizing and stimulating workers. Veteran nurses who had grown to accept the toxic culture and organizational problems in their work environments were suddenly energized and inspired. These nurses were asked to talk about what didn't work and what they thought would make it better. They were also invited to participate in helping implement those changes and given real authority to enforce compliance.

At one of these meetings, a nurse from a small community hospital in the Upper Peninsula, with a four-bed ICU, shared a story. An older woman with gray hair, who had probably been a nurse for more than twenty years, she said, "I've got to tell you, Dr. Pronovost, you have changed my hospital. We were using your checklist and one of the senior doctors came in and didn't wash his hands. So I said, 'You've got to go back and fix this.' And he responded, 'What do you mean, I have to go back and fix this? This is the way I put lines in.' I said, 'No, that is not the way you do it anymore. Dr. Pronovost says so and if you don't go do it right now I am going to page him and tell him.' The doctor asked me, 'Who is Dr. Pronovost?' And I said, 'He is the ICU doctor from Johns Hopkins and I am going to page him if you don't do it the right way.' And he said, 'I have seen his research; he is doing great work. No, no, I don't want you to do that. I'll do it your way.'"

At another one of our talks Chris got four hundred handheld mirrors and left them on the tables. When it was my turn to speak on stage I said, "Pick up that mirror and take a look at your image. In the reflection of that mirror is a leader who has an essential role in making care safer in Michigan and the world. We all have to accept that responsibility. Without each of you this is not going to happen. This is not my project; it is collectively your project."

Thanks to the informative and collaborative group calls and these inspirational face-to-face sessions, momentum continued to build. However, we did encounter significant tension with one hospital—the big and powerful University of Michigan Health System. University of Michigan is a great institution with great clinicians. The university president sat on the board of MHA and the clinicians were concerned that MHA had turned to Hopkins and not them to do this work. The association responded by telling them that Hopkins was the national leader in this kind of work. Perhaps not surprisingly, the University of Michigan was reluctant to commit all of its ICUs. The hospital had six adult ICUs at the time and only the medical ICU was in the program.

Even that ICU had come to us a bit tentatively. It wasn't until we were a couple of weeks into the project that the director of the medical ICU, Bob Hyzy, an associate professor of pulmonary critical care medicine, became a little curious. Because he liked the science behind our work he decided to put his toe in the water. I knew Bob from his research on lung disease and had a lot of respect for him as a clinician and researcher.

University of Michigan had been getting a lot of pressure from the MHA so Bob decided to join one of the calls to see what this was all about. He was impressed by our work but he wasn't convinced his ICU had significant problems with central line infections. I asked him to go look at his data. At our next meeting he admitted that infection rates were not where he wanted them to be.

I knew how important it was to get all of University of Michigan's ICUs on board, so I scheduled a lunch with Bob where I acknowledged that we were struggling with his hospital and sought his leadership. He went back to his colleagues and recruited the rest of the University of Michigan's ICUs to participate. As a result, University of Michigan achieved dramatic reductions, and Bob now leads the ongoing ICU collaborative for the Keystone Center.

Although we were successful at inspiring staff, we had a different set of challenges with the hospital CEOs. Unlike doctors and nurses, many CEOs are far removed from the practice of medicine. They do not experience the exhausting day-in, day-out, frontline struggle of trying to keep patients alive and well. And therefore they don't experience the importance of patient safety the way a clinician does. Yet we knew these executives wanted to make a difference and supported our mission.

One of my most profound lessons on how to energize management came at an MHA executive retreat on Mackinac Island. I was on stage addressing more than fifty CEOs and another hundred CFOs and COOs sitting at twenty large round tables. During a dinner meeting, I talked about the project and what we were doing to reduce infections. I shared with them the concept of Ohana, that we are a family and we have to guarantee safe care for all the people of Michigan. Most of the audience seemed rather bored.

I said, "We should not compete on safety. It's not about hospital against hospital, nor is it CEOs versus doctors or doctors versus nurses. We all have a moral obligation to work together to improve care for patients."

When I finished we had a question-and-answer session. One of the CEOs in the front stood up and said, "You know, Peter, everyone tells us that leadership is important, that leadership has to support this and lead the way, but can you tell me, what the hell does that mean? I need something concrete. I need specific direction. Tell me what I have to do. I am a busy CEO. I don't think in conceptual models, I think in actions. When I go back in my office on Monday what is it you want me to do?"

Perhaps because of the wine and cocktails or because this CEO made himself vulnerable, the discussion quickly opened up. Although these executives knew patient safety was an important topic and were fundamentally committed to doing the right thing, they did not have a clear strategy or plan for how to improve it. And until now, most had likely been afraid to say so.

One CEO said, "You do not get to be CEO without having answers to questions. Yet I do not have a clue what to do to improve safety. I am not comfortable admitting that."

I responded, "I am leading this project and I do not have all the answers, either. That is okay. What I do know is we have to set a goal of zero infections and work to realize it. We will work out the technical details together; what is important is your commitment to set a goal, measure progress, and work to achieve it. I understand this is difficult and you are busy. What if I made this easy for you? What if we were to send you one simple task for you to do each month, would that help?"

They liked the idea. Our first trial run came when we learned most of the hospitals used an antiseptic solution called Betadine to clean the skin prior to placing a central line. Although this was somewhat effective, a similar product called chorhexidine had been proven to be 50 percent more effective at reducing infections. Even though the two cost about the same, only 20 percent of the hospitals in Michigan stocked chlorhexidine in the kits they used to insert central lines.

We went to the doctors and nurses and encouraged them to change the antiseptic solutions in the kits used to place central lines, but the staff didn't know how to make this happen. Ironically no one we talked to had the authority or even had a clue how the hospital ordered its supplies. I figured that the CEOs could help us with this. So we sent all of the CEOs a memo asking them to make sure that, within one month, every hospital in the state stocked chorhexidine in their central line kits. I said that we would check back at the end of the month to see if they had done it. We had absolutely no formal authority over these CEOs. They did not have to comply; I was simply a physician from Maryland on temporary loan to their state. Yet in spite of this, in one month it was done. All of the hospitals had switched to using chlorhexidine when placing central lines. When the clinicians realized that their voices had been heard, that the CEOs got the job done, it only further cemented their commitment and trust in the project. The energy was palpable and when infection rates started to plummet, that excitement grew even bigger.

At this point everything seemed to be humming along, yet we were still very concerned about collecting accurate and complete data. I was constantly reminded of Sorrel King's simple question, "Is a child like Josie less likely to die?" Patients and their families are not interested in ideas, theories, or new safety programs; all they care about is results. They want to know that a hospital is in fact safer. Having complete data was the only way I could definitively answer that question.

Accurate and complete data speaks directly to our integrity as researchers, and my team viewed quality work as research. To do this work without solid data was nothing short of scientific misconduct. Frankly, much of the safety work that had been done to date, if viewed as research, would be seen as misconduct. Not necessarily out of bad intent but simply because the data was fatally flawed. Data was either missing or of poor quality and as a result, any conclusion that the project improved safety was suspect at best. I believe this is the principal reason many of these programs often failed to deliver safer care to patients. Most, if not all, of the groups working to improve health care were likely doing so with the best intentions, but if they couldn't point to numbers that clearly showed what they were doing worked, that it was actually saving lives, they couldn't tell the Sorrel Kings of the world that patients were safer because they didn't have the evidence.

Two months into studying the work at Michigan, our biggest fear had become a reality. We had 60 percent missing data—only 40 percent of our institutions were reporting results the way we had asked. With this much missing data it was impossible to validly conclude whether patients were safer. The only thing I could conclude was that we had no clue. It was heartbreaking. Ours was no different from the other quality improvement projects that claimed to be improving safety but had no real proof. I was devastated. We could not let this happen. It went against my training and everything we believed in. And worse yet, we knew it would guarantee our failure.

I called Chris and said, "This is unacceptable. We need to be accountable to the public. Tell all of the hospitals that they need to submit the required data or they are out of the project."

Chris said, "I am with you on this, Peter, but you need to know that this is not how quality is done in this country. Quality is a concept that has never been viewed as research or science. As long as hospitals are doing projects they think will make patients safer, they believe patients are safer."

I knew she was correct in her assessment, but I also knew that this was unacceptable. Quality without science and research is absurd. You can't make inferences that something works when you have 60 percent missing data. From a research perspective it's un-

ethical; it violates the principle code of conduct for scientific research. For years the safety community has made a distinction
between safety work and research. These experts basically take the
attitude that the means justify the ends—that safety work is a noble
pursuit regardless of the results. Therefore, unlike research, they
don't feel as if they need to measure results. The problem is, without solid data, improving safety is nothing more than a marketing
ploy with little or no substance. Patients deserve better. Considering that lives are at stake, it is almost shameful. If we do not have a
good measurement system, safety practices will likely continue to
fail and waste time and money. Even worse, patients will continue
to suffer and die. No one before us had required such robust measurement in patient safety. We felt it was our moral duty to make a
stand.

I didn't need to convince Chris; she already understood these
concepts. A career health care worker who worked her way up the
ladder though hard work, talent, and insight, she wanted to see real
change as much as I did. Chris knew that the reason Michigan hospitals were eager to work with us was because we did good science;
we had real results. What we needed was to somehow get hospitals
to understand the importance of good measurement and do whatever it takes to collect that data consistently. What they needed was
a little push.

So, with renewed strength and a clear purpose—quality data—
we talked to Spence Johnson, the president of the Michigan Hospital Association, and asked him if he would issue a memo to all of the
hospitals in our program encouraging them to reduce the amount of
missing data. If a hospital could not supply good data, we would ask
it to drop out of the program. Of course I didn't think that would be
necessary since I had full confidence that each hospital had the abil-

ity to produce complete data. It was just that nobody had ever called them out on their data quality and nobody ever encouraged them to do better. We wanted to reset the bar for what data quality means to quality improvement.

Spence understood, as we did, the need to know with confidence whether we had reduced infections, so he agreed to send the memo. Just as we had hoped, not a single hospital dropped out of the program. More importantly, the quantity of data jumped from 40 percent complete to 95 percent—an even higher success rate than we expected. Indeed, 5 percent missing data is as good or better than most well-funded randomized clinical trials that use a trained, paid data collector. This response further ignited my belief that clinicians in Michigan wanted to know whether they were improving care as much as we did. We were finally bringing safety and science together; we would finally have real proof that patients were going to be safer; we were making change happen.

The results were astonishing. Only three months after we started the study, the overall median rate of catheter-related bloodstream infection dropped from 2.7 infections per 1,000 catheter days to nearly zero. This means that at least half of the ICUs nearly eliminated these infections during this period. That rate stayed at zero for the entire eighteen months of the study. In fact, the rates were still staying the same four years later. Our work in nearly eliminating central line infection in Michigan saves an estimated two thousand lives and $200 million a year. Granted, these numbers for lives and dollars saved are estimated from published studies of how many people with these infections die and how much these infections cost, and as such are not precise. However, even if we are somewhere in the ballpark of these numbers, it is still profound.

What was even more inspiring was that these results came from applying our work to one problem in one unit. Imagine what might happen if we spread our work throughout the hospital to all systems and all levels of care? That was exactly what was happening back where it all started, at Hopkins.

# Chapter 6

W e'd come a long way since those early days in the Hopkins SICU and the WICU. And at each step along the way we learned. In the operating room we learned that our TRIP model needed more focus on culture, thus giving birth to CUSP. Similarly, working large-scale in Michigan necessitated the merging of TRIP and CUSP into the integrated CUSP model. It is this revised CUSP model that we began exporting to units outside the WICU and SICU. And just as we expected, we still had much to learn.

The most obvious units to tackle first were the four remaining adult ICUs—the medical intensive care unit (MICU), the neurosciences critical care unit (NCCU), the coronary care unit (CCU), and the cardiac surgical intensive care unit (CSICU).

Since these units were similar in many ways to the SICU and WICU, for the most part we had little trouble implementing CUSP. We were especially proud of the results from our central line checklist. Patients in the CSICU are some of the sickest we see in the hospital, especially heart transplant and lung transplant patients. And almost all of these patients need central lines. Yet the CSICU took what was a relatively high infection rate and all but eliminated it.

CUSP wasn't as big a hit, however, in the MICU. The MICU specializes in nonsurgical adult patients, the majority of whom have suffered heart problems, bleeding from stomach ulcers, or drug overdoses or have respiratory, kidney, or liver disease. What separates the MICU from the rest of Hopkins' ICUs is that it falls under the Department of Medicine, whereas the rest of the ICUs are in the departments of Surgery and Anesthesiology and Critical Care Medicine. This means the MICU is outside of my direct sphere of influence. Like most hospitals, the hierarchy at Hopkins is divided along department lines. Doctors within the Department of Medicine are much more likely to cooperate with their own than with a doctor from the Department of Anesthesiology and Critical Care Medicine, like me.

Sometimes conflicts among doctors are open and direct, but most of the time they are shrouded in passive-aggressive behavior. I heard through the grapevine that many of the MICU doctors didn't trust our results, didn't think that the daily goals reduced length of stay and errors, and didn't believe we could reduce bloodstream infections. Even though the data was collected independently by hospital epidemiology staff, MICU doctors were skeptical.

In many ways this was understandable. The Department of Medicine is one of the most conservative departments at Hopkins, making it especially resistant to change. This conservatism is not unfounded. This legendary department is one of the oldest in the hospital and has produced many of the world's leading doctors and researchers. As such, its members are some of the most evidence-dedicated, scholarly physicians in the hospital. Obviously we had somehow failed to present clear, indisputable, science-based evidence proving that CUSP was worth the effort. I welcomed and valued the skepticism. Patient safety measures need to be evidence based. If we're going to ask doctors to change what they do, we better have data that proves, without a doubt, that patients will be better off as a result of this change and will not suffer unintentional harm.

By this point, I had learned that if there is an elephant in the room, you have to talk about it (or in my case sometimes even sit on it). If MICU doctors had concerns about my work it was better to face this doubt head-on. It can be risky, and often unpleasant, but I had grown accustomed to catching heat for my work. Rather than push back, I try to listen. I put on my Kevlar vest and absorb the blows. What protects me is the sincere belief that the work, and everything we do in medicine, is about the patient. If I ever let that focus change from patient centered to Pronovost centered, I knew I would lose the support of my fellow physicians.

This is not the first time I had experienced resistance from the Department of Medicine. I remember meeting once with the chief residents and junior faculty from the entire department to explain daily goals and how the system could be implemented in their department. The meeting took place in a large, wood-paneled conference room surrounded by pictures of prior giants in medicine. I talked about the evidence behind our work, the benefits and potential risk, and made it clear that patients would benefit greatly from having nurses and doctors do rounds together and use our daily goals tool. I asked for input on how this concept would need to be modified to fit a medical floor.

The chief residents thought I was from Mars. Their culture was very physician centered and they could not understand why nurses would need to participate in rounds with them. They were physicians, doing physician things; they alone made the decisions.

I responded by saying, "I understand you need to make decisions, yet you will make wiser decisions with diverse and independent input. The nurses are with the patients much more than you are, they see things you do not, and you will make better decisions if you incorporate what they say. Who do you think is going to implement all the plans you make? Nurses. It seems to me that it would be much more effective and efficient and safer for patients if nurses heard the plan and commented on it and everyone was clear about what to do."

I might as well have been talking Swahili, because it was blatantly obvious that we did not connect. The physicians rejected my science of safety in favor of the antiquated autonomous physician model. I was not surprised. The wood paneling and the faces on the old paintings that hung on those walls reflected an era when that model made sense. And change is not easy. I left frustrated. I was convinced that using daily goals with an interdisciplinary care team is a powerful patient safety tool. How could we get doctors to see the light? Until culture changed, we would likely remain in the dark.

When I met with MICU doctors I was better prepared. I brought along the hard data from our work in Michigan and Hopkins. I asked the doctors if they believed the current communication and safety standards in the Department of Medicine were as good as they could be. If not, why not give our program a try? The risks were clearly minimal compared to the benefits. After considerable cajoling, reducing the actual losses, dispelling the perceived losses, and being sensitive to tender egos, I somehow managed to get the message through. And once these doctors got it, once the light went on, they not only adopted the central line checklist, they embraced CUSP full-on. Doctors are, at the core, scientists. Once they get something, once they understand and believe the science, they are in.

Unlike the physicians, the MICU nurses were immediately on

board. One of these nurses who was a real CUSP champion was Dana Moore, a clinical nurse specialist who is passionate about safety. We use the term "CUSP champion" to describe people who embrace CUSP and become true leaders. Although it was important to get the doctors on board, most of these CUSP initiatives don't even get off the ground without a strong nurse leader who is willing to devote four to eight hours a week toward this work.

The MICU effort also couldn't have made it without a strong executive member. In this case, the vice president of Human Resources at Johns Hopkins Hospital and Health System, Pamela Paulk, stepped up to the plate. Pamela's experience made her a natural for working with staff-related issues. Pamela is a compassionate and progressive executive and was a CUSP champion from the get-go. Pamela's kindness and compassion go well above the call of duty. (Only just recently she decided to donate one of her kidneys to a man who works on the Hopkins maintenance staff. Her motivation? She knew the man was sick and felt it was the right thing to do.)

One of the first problems the team addressed was whether or not they should keep patients sedated when they are on ventilators. To date they had been keeping these patients sedated to benefit nurses (it made these patients easier to care for) and a perceived benefit to patients (staff assumed the patients with a breathing tube stuck in their throat would be more comfortable sedated than if they were conscious).

Dale Needham, one of the MICU doctors working on our safety team, questioned this logic. Dale not only showed that patients do better with less sedation, but he actually started to get these patients (on breathing machines with tubes in their throats) walking and exercising. Once he put this theory into action, no one argued that it was much more beneficial to the healing process to have these patients up and moving around than it was to have them bedridden and unconscious.

Another problem the CUSP team tackled was a serious issue related to pain medication. Dana and her team (along with the rest of the hospital and the world) had a long-standing problem with accidentally overdosing patients with narcotics. When a patient becomes agitated, it's sometimes necessary to increase his or her sedation medication—usually a narcotic. Agitated patients often pull out catheters and breathing tubes or can otherwise harm themselves.

When this happened, typically a nurse would increase the setting on the medication pump used to deliver the sedation medication. After about one or two minutes, the nurse would turn it back down to its prescribed setting. However, as is common in the busy world of medicine, a nurse can easily be called away for an emergency and forget to lower the setting. When this happens, the patient receives an overdose. For the most part, patients do not suffer harm, but overdoses can be dangerous and can even kill. Large doses of narcotics can lower blood pressure to dangerous levels, harming a patient's organs. Most importantly, narcotics can also suppress and even stop a patient's breathing, which is dangerous for patients not on ventilators. If you stop breathing, you will die.

The unit had four instances of overdose in the two years prior to implementing our CUSP program, none of them fatal. Three of these patients were not harmed because, like most of the patients in the MICU, they were on breathing machines. However, one of these patients was not on a breathing machine and might have died, if not for the fact that he had a high tolerance for narcotics. In essence, the staff got lucky. In a strange irony, the patient was a heroin addict and therefore tolerant to high doses of narcotics—his addiction probably saved his life. Still, luck is not the way we want to run a hospital. Errors like these were too close for comfort—it was only a matter of time before our luck ran out.

"Before CUSP came along we tried a lot of little fixes," says Dana. "Instead of turning up the machine, we asked the nurse to go and get an ampoule of medication and physically inject it."

This reduced the chance of medication pump errors but opened up other risks. Some ampoules contain very high and very concentrated doses of narcotics while others have watered-down doses. It is actually common for patients to get drug overdoses when nurses don't realize they are using a concentrated drug. Secondly, when a patient is agitated you often don't want to leave them unattended for long, or even at all. And it can take a while to punch in the security code and retrieve the needed drug from the medication locker.

Dana said the unit had also tried to have nurses wait by the bedside until the patient had received the full extra dose and then turn the machine back down. They also tried having nurses regularly check the pumps to make sure they were at a normal setting. Unfortunately, these tactics assume that people will not make errors. Since we are human and fallible by nature, these improvements were generally ineffective.

What we often find is that quick fixes like these may reduce some risks but will inevitably introduce new ones. If you do not anticipate and protect against these new risks, you could actually make things worse. If we want to make wise decisions that reduce rather than enhance harm to patients, safety has to be rooted in science and evidence—you need to pilot test and evaluate your intervention.

A solution to the problem they were having with medication pumps came out of one of the CUSP meetings when a nurse told us about safe pumps that had a built-in timer that would automatically return medication levels back to normal after they had been

increased. We all agreed that this was the best solution to this issue and our executive pulled some strings to get money to purchase
them. We exchanged all our old medication pumps on the MICU
for safe pumps and measured the results. The team counted the frequency and type of medication errors before and after the introduction of the new pumps, using clear and rigorous definitions. The
results? These medication errors were virtually eliminated. In fact,
the new pumps are so successful in improving safety they are now
standard issue in all units across the hospital.

This is a great example of the value of executive involvement—
connecting a decision maker with a clinical need. Getting new
equipment costs money, and money is scarce and political. Often
many layers are involved in making a request and months or years
between recognizing a need and receiving money to buy the needed
equipment. CUSP streamlines that process. Just as in Michigan,
when CEOs quickly delivered the chlorhexidine we requested, executives like Pamela know exactly what to do and who to call to
fast-lane change.

Executives not only have power to make change and allocate
money but they also exercise influence over physicians. For example,
when we gave nurses the pager numbers of top executives in the
SICU, it was the magic ingredient that helped encourage the doctors to listen to the nurses. Similarly if doctors know an executive is
going to attend a CUSP meeting, you can be sure they are going to
do their best to be there. Executives also offer a unique perspective,
since they are often the only nonclinicians in the room. They can
provide a certain type of clarity that is often missing when a group of
similarly minded people gets together to problem-solve.

It clearly takes all CUSP team members working together to
achieve success. When physicians do not lend support to the pro-

gram it is very difficult or impossible to make change happen, since the rest of the team ultimately takes their orders from the doctors. Also doctors, with their knowledge of medicine, have to be involved in CUSP so the team can design interventions that are effective and that all the physicians on the team will trust and use. Doctors also see different errors than staff—for example, errors that involve diagnosis and treatment rather than the day-to-day workings of the unit.

Similarly, nurses also play a huge role in making CUSP successful. Nurses often spend the most time both with patient and in the unit and, therefore, often have a tremendous amount of knowledge regarding safety issues. After solutions are identified, it's often up to the nurses to put the initiatives into action, which inevitably means additional work. Clearly, if you did not have nurses on board, CUSP wouldn't even get off the ground.

As we expanded CUSP to different units in the hospital, it became clear we were going to need help managing this project. After our success in Michigan, our research team was already up to its ears trying to spread CUSP into other states. We clearly needed dedicated people in the hospital who could focus primarily on this Hopkins work. Luckily our top executives recognized this need and allocated some funding to support a Center for Innovation in Quality Patient Care and appointed me as its medical director and Chip Davis as executive director. Chip and I have been working together for several years to improve quality and safety. Using some of the money from the center's budget, we were able to hire Lori Paine to head up patient safety and lead the Hopkins CUSP efforts. Lori is a career nurse who has strong administrative credentials and a good amount of experience in patient safety work at Hopkins. Lori would lead a group of CUSP coaches and champions who, like her, would be responsible for coaching and training CUSP teams.

This funding also helped us build a Web-based error reporting system called the Patient Safety Net (PSN). This hospitalwide computer system helps with our safety work by allowing staff to anonymously report safety issues throughout the hospital. We currently get nearly fifteen thousand Hopkins error reports annually.

Since improving safety is a science, we also hired several experts who understand the way organizations are structured and how people and systems interact. These professionals are tasked with analyzing dysfunctional systems and fixing them. The tools they use were developed in industry, to reduce variation and waste in processes, and have since been imported into health care. Since our work is all about rooting out bad systems, these people have been invaluable. The hospital president, Ron Peterson, gave us the support we needed on this.

"The premise that doctors are not trained to be systems engineers is a fundamental truth. We are dealing with complicated processes that involve multiple people across departmental lines. It is very useful for us to introduce into the hospital environment people who are trained differently. I think we have benefited greatly both in terms of patient safety but also in terms of improving efficiency of our operations by introducing these different kinds of skill sets," says Ron Peterson.

We are fortunate that our hospital leadership recognized the importance of investing resources in patient safety. Unfortunately, few hospitals have made these types of investments; few have the capital to do so. Health care must develop mechanisms for improving the delivery and the quality of health services, and for reducing costs. Unfortunately, the financial rewards from these improvements often do not go directly to the hospital but to the insurer. Without having a clear profit gain to point to, it is not always easy to get management on board. That being said, many CFOs, including our own, are beginning to see that, although the short-term financial gain of patient safety might be murky, the long-term financial gain is clear.

One of the units Lori tackled with her new team was Weinberg-4C. These nurses and doctors take care of surgical patients from the Weinberg operating room after the patient has left the WICU. When Weinberg-4C first approached us with an interest in CUSP, staff turnover was high (around 20 percent per year), moral was low, conflicts between physicians and nurses were common, and mistakes from poor communication occurred frequently.

Luckily some of the residents in Weinberg-4C had been in the WICU, had learned the science of safety, had used the daily goals, understood good teamwork, and wanted to bring those essentials to the unit. Equally, nurse manager Joanne Timmel and the director of surgical nursing, Deborah Baker, knew of CUSP and its impact on rounds and were eager to take it on. I decided to be the executive for this unit for a couple of reasons. First, I wanted to see firsthand how CUSP worked outside the ICU. Second, my work in the WICU had given me a unique sensitivity to the difficulties we might have getting surgeons on board with CUSP.

We launched the program by giving the science of safety talk. I delivered it on a cold, rainy evening to a room full of nurses—the smells of pepperoni pizza, chocolate chip cookies, and Coke filled the room. Just as I suspected, no physicians attended. But nevertheless we continued. I asked the nurses if they knew how the next patient would be harmed. All hands went up. One nurse told the story of how she once had a surgical patient who was developing septic shock before her eyes—this is when a patient has a bloodstream infection so severe it is attacking and shutting down organs. Yet the patient was not on antibiotics, the patient was not getting the treatments he needed, the patient had not been sent to the ICU, where the nurse felt he belonged, and the situation was desperate.

Worse yet, the nurse was forced to play phone tag, paging one doctor who told her he was not on call and another who said he was not on service. The nurse became tearful telling her story. I could feel her frustration and pain. She felt helpless. It is a horrible feeling to be standing before a patient, watching him or her die, knowing it's your job to try to prevent it, but not being able to get anyone to listen. The nurse finally got hold of a surgeon who was in the operating room. Hours went by, and although the patient eventually went to the ICU he subsequently died from the overwhelming infection.

After listening to that powerful story I handed out the CUSP questionnaire that asked how the next patient would be harmed and what could we do about it. When we received the questionnaires back, we found that 80 percent of the nurses said communication was the biggest problem. (This is roughly the response we get in every unit.) In particular the nurses uniformly said they had no clue about plans of care—what the doctors planned to do, when the patient was going home, what was needed to make that happen—and no understanding of how they could help. In short, there was no real care team; this was a dysfunctional unit.

Luckily we had a potential cure for this problem—the daily goals tool. If we could get the entire team to do rounds together, we were confident everyone would be clear on each patient's daily plan of care. However, we soon learned we faced challenges in this unit that would make implementing daily goals much more difficult here than it was in the ICU.

Daily goals worked well in the ICU because all the patients were under the same care team. Furthermore, this team—the attending, residents, nurses, and associated staff—conducted rounds on all patients in the unit at the same time every day. On the medical and surgical floors, patients were cared for by a variety of doctors from different "services"—plastic surgery, surgical oncology, orthopedic surgery, general surgery, and others. So, in addition to the unit-based team—the nurses and staff that work on that unit—there were often many service-based teams, treating each different type of patient. This made communication and teamwork very difficult and daily goals next to impossible. As many as ten or twelve service teams might be making rounds anytime between six and seven a.m. Because each floor nurse cared for patients that belonged to a number of services, doing separate rounds with each of these doctors was impossible. Also, these physicians had patients distributed throughout the hospital so they typically didn't spend much time on the unit, making communication that much more difficult.

It was painfully clear we were going to have to make some serious changes if we wanted to apply daily goals to Weinberg-4C. And changes were going to require physician support. Luckily one of the doctors on the CUSP team was the surgeon in charge of the surgical oncology service, Dr. Richard Schulick. I have known Rich since medical school at Hopkins. He is an excellent surgeon with great communication and team skills who has been helping lead the charge to improve hospital culture. I called him and said that I wanted to try making rounds with the nurses and doing daily goals. He had seen the benefits of doing this in the WICU and agreed to help make this happen.

At our next CUSP meeting we discussed the problem. The nurses quickly raised the issue that daily goals at rounds was not possible, given that so many different services admitted patients to the unit. I suggested that we try to group patients of a specific service together in the unit so there could be more of a team, something we call cohorting. Joanne was a strong proponent of this idea. In essence, by cohorting patients we could create the team structure that we had in the ICU. We could not do this with all the services in the Weinberg-4C unit, so we chose the largest, which was the service run by Rich. He and his residents treated patients who had surgery primarily for pancreatic cancer. Grouping his patients together would not only help to include the nurses on rounds, but also help those nurses develop expertise in managing a specific patient group.

The reason the unit didn't cohort patients was because the administration believed that it was more efficient to put a new patient in the first available bed. That meant that whenever a bed was empty and there was a patient who needed it, they would put that patient in that bed regardless of whether there were any other patients nearby that had the same illness and physicians or whether the nurses there were skilled in caring for that type of patient. That meant doctors were forced to travel all over the hospital to see their patients, which was not only highly inefficient, but it created many more patient safety issues. And it virtually precluded nurses being part of a care team. This method of bed distribution is the generally accepted model in U.S. hospitals—although nobody had actually done a scientific study to prove it works. It's also a classic example of fixing one problem and creating another. While it is true patients get into beds faster using the old system (and thus may alleviate emergency room crowding), these patients likely suffer more complications as a result of having uncoordinated care plans and therefore suffer longer hospital stays.

When I explained the plan about cohorting patients so we could invite nurses on rounds, Rich thought it was a good idea. He strongly favored trying it and believed patient safety would improve. His only stipulations were that he wanted to be sure that the time needed for his residents to do rounds wasn't increased, and he wanted the residents to measure this themselves. I agreed on measurement but I did not think the surgeons should do it. Self-monitoring is inaccurate, subjective, and not at all scientific. I suggested that a better measure would be to monitor the number of pages the residents received. He agreed.

I chose this form of measurement because it was objective and clearly defined, and it spoke to the real problem—communication. Fewer pages would tell us communication had improved; the same number or more pages would tell us it hadn't. Besides providing us with a measure of success, getting fewer pages would also give doctors and nurses more time for other work and free them from the irritation of excessive pages, which only further erodes teamwork.

With Rich on board I went to the director of surgical nursing, Deborah Baker, and asked her if we could consider cohorting Rich's patients on the floor. I explained to her the reasoning behind this move, and Deb, being a strong supporter of safety efforts, agreed. The group wouldn't include all patients admitted to Weinberg-4C, since there were more beds than Rich had patients, but at least we could cohort Rich's patients and test to see if it worked.

We then set out to draft a daily goals form. Like all checklists, it needed to be adapted to fit the specific culture and context in which it was applied. The daily goals form we used in the ICU would not work here on the floor. In the ICU, patients were sicker and needed more daily procedures, so we really needed one separate form per patient. On the floor, we realized that a single sheet for each patient was both excessive and impractical. Also, in spite of our efforts to cohort we still had a number of services on the floor and couldn't always guarantee that individual bedside nurses would be free to make rounds with us. So we decided to have the nurse in charge of the floor do the rounds with the team. We created one daily goals sheet for the unit and made it the charge nurse's job to fill it out. The form listed each patient, the anticipated discharge date, what needed to happen for the patient to be discharged (for example, obtaining a social work consult or arranging home nursing), what goals the staff had for the patient that day, and the patient's poten tial safety risks.

After implementing our revised daily goals sheet, the number of pages the doctors received went from sixty-four per day to two. Both nurses and physicians saw it as a clear improvement. The word spread and soon and many other surgeons approached Deb to ask if their patients could be cohorted.

The second issue we addressed was the plastic surgery service. Its residents were so overworked that patients were not getting the level of care they needed. This is a common problem throughout the hospital and the nation. These surgeons are often in the operating room and the nurses have no one to call when their patients become sick. During CUSP meetings nurses, often in tears, told me horrible stories of being at the bedside of a deteriorating patient, someone who needed urgent attention, and calling the plastic surgery resident only to learn he or she was in the operating room and could not leave. It's not that they didn't care, they cared deeply, but it was a systemic problem; they had to stay in the operating room. One nurse told how she had a patient with diabetes who had a dangerously high blood sugar level. After the plastic surgery resident did not respond, the nurse paged the endocrinology fellow who had been consulting on the patient to evaluate and treat high blood sugar. The fellow came and treated the patient—a perfectly appropriate thing to do. Yet when the resident came out of the operating room later that evening, he exploded at the nurse, verbally abused her, and demanded that the charge nurse submit an incident report on her for inappropriately calling another doctor.

Surgeons are known for these kinds of outbursts. Anyone who has worked in a hospital knows doctors often throw tantrums, act like spoiled children, and even verbally assault nurses. However, the fact remains, surgeons are grossly overworked, often sleep deprived, and under extreme pressure to perform flawlessly. And this kind of behavior, although unacceptable, is in many ways predictable. Hospitals don't provide training for these doctors to deal with this kind of stress. Furthermore, the hours and lifestyle of this work can lead to poor health and exhaustion. When you place a person who is overworked, hungry, and tired into a stressful, high-stakes conflict, the predictable result is aggression. Sleep deprivation likely plays a major role. It has been proven that after twenty-four hours without sleep, people function as though they are legally drunk. At thirty-six hours they function like a paranoid schizophrenic and their emotions rule over logic. Most surgeons work those long hours on a regular basis, so it's not surprising they can get irritable and aggressive.

The solution Weinberg-4C came up with to help alleviate the pressure on our plastic surgery residents and provide better care for the patients was to hire nurse practitioners. These staff members have the skill level to identify when a patient is deteriorating and the power to summon help. They have the training to make decisions about a patient's care plan and can write orders for therapy. But although these professionals are easier to hire (nurse practitioners don't cost as much as physicians), hiring new staff still costs money and budgets are always an issue.

However, thanks to support from the chair of surgery, and some heavy lobbying that included data from incident reports and real stories of overworked residents and of patients who were placed in danger because residents were in the operating room, the department hired a nurse practitioner for the plastic surgery division. We also stipulated that this person's job was to be on the floor, answering pages and responding to emergencies—not in the operating room. Moreover, he or she would be unit based. This was a novel concept outside the ICU. Most nurse practitioners and residents are service based and roam multiple units. We wanted to create the teamlike atmosphere we had in the ICU. Having a nurse practitioner who never left the unit would help create this atmosphere.

We also purchased some wireless monitors that would notify the nurse practitioner directly whenever a patient was not doing well. This mitigated a significant safety issue. During CUSP meetings the staff complained that there were dead zones in the unit where they could not send or receive pages. These occur for a variety of reasons throughout the hospital and pose huge risks. Even worse, there is no warning system indicating that the page sent did not go through. A nurse could think that he or she had sent an urgent page to a physician, then wait for a response, only to find it was never sent, wasting valuable time that could save a life. Though a better fix would have been to correct the dead spots, it was not technically possible at the time and wireless monitors proved to be an easier, more practical, and equally effective solution.

The impact of CUSP on Weinberg-4C was profound. Staff turnover went from 20 percent to nearly zero, culture and teamwork scores improved dramatically, nurse satisfaction and surgeon satisfaction improved, and length of stay for patients was reduced. It only further proves how culture and systems are interdependent—changing one changes the other. When the changes are positive, it is energizing. When negative, it feels like an organizational death spiral that demoralizes the entire team.

Next on deck was the medical primary care unit, MPCU-4. MPCU-4 is for nonsurgical patients who are not sick enough to be in an ICU but not quite well enough to stay on a regular hospital floor. The executive chosen to lead this CUSP group was the chief financial officer of the Johns Hopkins Health System, Ronald Werthman. CFOs are often thought to be the least passionate about hospital work and patient care because they are so wrapped up in the money end of health care. Often called the "bean counters," it's their job to keep an eye on the bottom line. The margins in hospitals are very small and the CFO has to rigorously manage costs to keep these small margins positive. In order to be effective, CFOs have to be practical, not emotional, when it comes to cutting jobs and hacking away unprofitable services. Since the return on investment for patient safety work is hard to measure (these benefits often occur in the future and likely get passed on to insurers), and safety programs usually require investments, one might think a CFO might be less than enthusiastic about investing in patient safety over, say, hiring a new clinician who can generate revenue.

Of course, like so many generalizations, this proved to be totally false. Ron turned out to be one of our best advocates for patient safety, embracing his new role as CUSP executive. Before he even got started working with Lori and her team, he spent a day shadowing a nurse just so he could better understand the daily workings of the unit. Most executives, or for that matter most anyone who isn't a nurse or doctor, might not get anywhere near as deeply involved. As Lori so aptly says, "They would probably be grossed out by all the blood and bodily fluids associated with daily nursing care." But Ron saw the importance of seeing hospital work through a different lens and taking the time to understand the work. It wasn't the first or the last time Ron shadowed doctors and nurses in their work. "It gives me a perspective that I didn't have. It gives me a better understanding of what these nurses and doctors do during the day and some of the things they go through," he says.

What's really exciting about this work is it is not about the specific program or even CUSP. It is about people. As I say over and over, and will continue to say, health care workers want to do good work. It's human nature to want to excel, to shine, and to be recognized. Health care self-selects these people, identifying those who have a particularly strong desire to take care of others—it's what attracts us to the field. Unfortunately, that energy, that desire to do good is often beaten out of clinicians by years of bad culture in the workplace. CUSP reawakens and cultivates that energy, giving it a chance to thrive and bloom.

One of the first problems the team addressed in MPCU-4 was central line maintenance. This unit had already adopted the checklist for placing central line catheters, and although they had greatly reduced the infection rates on the unit, infections had not been eliminated. The CUSP team got together to study this issue and came up with some interesting observations. Patients generally stay much longer in the MPCU-4 than they do in the ICU. Given this extended stay many of these patients have a central line in for a much longer period of time. These central line catheters are connected to a secondary long tube that runs to a medication pump that delivers drugs to the patient. Studies have shown that the secondary tube needs to be replaced every three days because of a risk that it will spread an infection to the patient. Each tube is labeled with a little sticker that has a date on it. When that date is three days old, the nurse is supposed to change it out. However, at one of our CUSP meetings, one of the nurses pointed out that many of these tubes were often left in past the expiration date, putting patients a greater risk of developing bloodstream infections. To confirm this, the unit ran a test and found out that the tubes were being replaced on schedule only 30 percent of the time.

So the CUSP team sat down and brainstormed on how to fix this problem and came up with a bright idea. The team surmised that the reason tubes were not being changed on time was because nurses had to look at the date on the tube, quickly do the math, and figure out if three days had passed. This might not seem difficult, but given the hectic pace of the hospital and all the other things nurses have to monitor and the dates they have to remember, it was a likely place for error.

So the MPCU-4 CUSP team came up with a better system. Instead of labeling a tube with the date when it was new, they decided to use the date when the tube needed to be replaced. That way the nurse could immediately see if it was old or not. Also the team decided to color-code the stickers according to the day of the week. This made it more visible and thus even easier. On a given day, all the pink tubes needed to be replaced or the green ones or the blue ones. To further reduce the risk for an error, the team created a chart that told nurses the colors for each day of the week. The chart was posted on the wall of the unit and the rate of error dropped to nearly zero. Problem fixed.

Another problem the team identified had to do with alarm fatigue. Each patient in this unit has a machine that monitors vital signs—heart rate, blood pressure, temperature, oxygen level in the blood, and breathing rate. If one of these levels is either too high or too low an alarm goes off, alerting a clinician that the patient is potentially in danger. When an alarm goes off and the patient is not in danger, it is called a false alarm. With fifteen patients on the unit, false alarms were frequent—producing what is known in hospitals as alarm fatigue. Alarm fatigue is when nurses, responding to false alarms, are constantly drawn away from other patients, or worse yet they get so used to these alarms they don't hear them or don't respond to them. Alarm fatigue puts all patients in the unit at risk and wastes the staff's precious time.

To alleviate this problem, some nurses were changing either the upper or lower alarm settings to reduce false alarms. It may sound like a reasonable solution but unless a solution is approached scientifically it can cause more harm than good. Such was the case here.

In one instance a nurse moved the upper threshold of a patient's heart rate monitor higher to reduce the number of false alarms the unit was getting. The patient had a high heart rate because his heart was not working efficiently. Because of this condition, moving his upper threshold on the monitor did not put the patient in danger. However, what did put the patient in danger was that the nurse didn't adjust his lower limit accordingly, leaving the patient with a rather large gap between the upper and lower alarm settings. His heart rate suddenly dropped from 150 to 60 beats per minute, which is dangerous for a person in his condition and should have set off an alarm. But no alarm sounded, a nurse was not summoned, and the patient went into heart failure and almost died.

This near death sent a shock wave across the unit. Nurses and doctors are affected deeply when a patient under their care almost dies. Guilt-ridden thoughts of "What could I have done?" and "What did I do wrong?" linger long after the event. Luckily there was a CUSP team in place to help them deal with this tragedy. A growing part of our work in safety is to support staff who make errors—especially errors that harm patients. These take a tremendous toll on them.

When the CUSP team discussed this issue they approached it, naturally, from a clinical perspective since they were almost all clinicians. Ron, the only nonclinician in the room, listened intently and, when it seemed appropriate, gave the perspective of a person who does not provide direct care for patients, but who works with numbers and data. This is one of the biggest contributions a senior executive can offer a CUSP team—a new perspective.

"When we first looked into this issue we could not find much in the medical literature about these alarms," Ron later said. "I suggested we get clinical engineering down to the unit to pull data off of the machine that was monitoring this patient. In my job we are constantly analyzing data. You cannot function on an anecdote. To run a place as large and complex as Hopkins you have to understand your data."

The team had no idea how to get this data, but Ron did. Or at least he knew who had the technical expertise. He called clinical engineering and they were on the unit the following day. Clinical engineering pulled the numbers and the team found that the patient's alarm had been going off every three seconds. It was no wonder the staff had alarm fatigue.

The old solution to a problem like this might have been to tell people to "try harder, to be more vigilant." The administration might have even put in some kind of penalty that it hoped would motivate clinicians to respond to every alarm and not change the threshold settings. But these quick fixes don't take into account human nature and human fallibility and therefore do not work.

Ron came up with a different solution. He contacted the vendor and learned that most of the staff had not been properly trained to operate these machines and the associated alarms; specifically, they were not setting the ranges correctly, which was resulting in a lot of false alarms. So he had the vendor, who manufactured the alarms, train the nurses so they better understood the features and limitations of the machines. Nurses then evaluated each patient and set the alarms according to that patient's particular risks and physiology. If the patient had a high resting heart rate, clinicians set both the upper and the lower limits on the high side; conversely, if the patient had a low heart rate, clinicians set them lower. As a result of this effort, false alarms dropped by 40 percent. In fact this was so successful, it was implemented across the hospital. It might sound very simple, and indeed sometimes the best solutions are. That is not to say we solved the problem of false alarms; we have not. They are an enormous problem throughout health care and will likely require a manufacturing solution. Still we made it better.

The final problem the CUSP team addressed in MPCU-4 were the handoffs—when a patient moves from one unit to another, in this case from the WICU to the MPCU-4. Handoffs are an excellent opportunity for the new care team members to learn everything they need to know about a patient from the previous care team. Unfortunately this was not always happening. People get busy and information is lost because there is no clear system to prevent these errors. Usually vital information is just scribbled on a piece of paper in what is often illegible handwriting. So the team created a handoff form. Now the new team knows what kind of issues this patient might have had in the ICU, such as the appropriate ranges for his alarm settings, as well as a wide variety of additional important information regarding the patient's care.

These CUSP initiatives did a lot to improve a number of identified problems in MPCU-4 as well as in the other units. They im-

proved teamwork, communication, and the general atmosphere of
the unit. But not all units have bad culture; in fact, some units we
visited already had excellent teamwork thanks to the independent
hard work of doctors and nurses. One of these units, our inpatient
AIDS clinic, Osler-8, had such good culture and teamwork scores,
Lori told the nurse manager, Sondra Garlic, "You already have it
going on, and probably didn't even need CUSP." Sondra replied,
"Thanks, but I know we can do it better."

Sondra and her team had worked hard to improve their unit; it
was important to them. In CUSP they saw an opportunity to expand on that good work. They also saw an opportunity to learn from
mistakes and to have an executive join their team, which helps a
unit address issues that are difficult to conquer with good culture
alone. Sometimes a little institutional muscle goes a long way. In
this case the executive was Richard Grossi, the CFO of Johns Hopkins Medicine, the organization that includes the medical school
and hospitals. Not a bad person to have on your side, especially if
you want to spend a little money.

At the first CUSP meeting, Osler-8 staff identified a number
of problems that needed attention. One issue that quickly rose to
the top of everyone's list was crowding in the semiprivate rooms.
Osler-8 is in an old part of the hospital and the semiprivate rooms
are a tiny twelve by twelve feet. Worse yet, the limited floor space in
these rooms had to accommodate two large hospital beds; two patient walkers; two cumbersome IV poles, each with a many-legged
stand; three trash cans (one for infectious, two for noninfectious
waste); two portable monitors; and a portable suction unit.

With all this extra equipment, there was very little empty
space to maneuver in these rooms, which put these patients at
risk since AIDS patients are prone to falling. AIDS patients can

have psychiatric and neurological issues that affect balance and judgment. Further compounding this issue, they often get better physically before they are better mentally, which makes them physically mobile while their ability to judge space and distance is still compromised. A crowded, cluttered room represents an enormous challenge to these patients. As a result they had a high fall rate in this unit.

The team brainstormed and came up with a viable, affordable solution. Thanks to help from Rich, they were able to get hospital maintenance to redesign the rooms so the suction machines and vital sign monitors were built into the walls and no longer took up floor space. The unit also eliminated the extra trash can for noninfectious waste. These initiatives alone lowered the unit's fall rate from five per month to two per month.

Sondra said one of the keys to the success in her unit was that everyone participated in the CUSP meetings. "The food service was not part of the problem but they offered to change the rate at which they picked up trays as a way to reduce clutter and help with fall rate. They could have ignored our problem but in the spirit of teamwork they became interested and tried to do what they could to help."

A second problem they encountered involved community-borne blood infections. Patients were bringing infections into the unit from the outside and these infections were spreading to other patients. For example, a staph infection (such as MRSA), is a challenge for a healthy person to battle, but for someone with AIDS, it can be life threatening. It often took three days or more before staff discovered that a patient was carrying an infection. By that time, the infection could have already spread. So the staff started testing patients when they first arrived and again when they left the unit.

They also kept one room empty so that the unit could isolate an infected patient.

"Up until we started testing patients upon arrival, we were being blamed for infecting these patients. We were putting a lot of energy into trying to keep things clean and trying to pinpoint the source of the infections on the unit," says Sondra. "Once we understood that these were not hospital-based infections but were actually coming in from the community, we had a better chance to fight them and to stop them from spreading."

Another project the Osler-8 unit worked on was hand washing—specifically, using the Purell dispensers whenever a clinician entered and left a patient's room. This was a large and well-run hospitalwide initiative, but the team believed they could improve on these efforts by having their own program. Indeed, many of the CUSP teams supplemented hospitalwide programs with their own ideas. The Osler-8 team decided to choose a secret observer who at the end of the day would identify staff who did excellent hand washing and put a flyer on the wall citing this person for his or her good work. At the end of the month whoever had his or her name on the wall the most frequently received a twenty-five-dollar gift certificate.

"We would reveal not only who was the best for the day, but also people who were close or did a pretty good job. Anyone who did well would get recognized—everyone was included on the floor: docs, social workers, et cetera," says Sondra.

These ideas might seem simple and obvious. But without a system in place that allows nurses and doctors to discuss new ideas and put them into action, without an executive to put muscle behind these initiatives and cut through red tape and get whatever small funding they need, these things never happen. Without support, many good ideas never get off the ground, which only further frustrates staff—a frustration that lowers morale and job satisfaction and only further endangers patients' safety.

The CUSP teams also learn from each other. Lori coordinates a monthly lunch with the CUSP leaders during which they discuss what interventions were effective. They share what each unit has learned and discuss how to further build capacity to improve safety.

In total we have exported CUSP to roughly a third of the units in the hospital and that number keeps growing.

With all this great work and experience behind us, and our constantly evolving and improving CUSP model, we were ready for the next step—taking our central line infection program across the nation. It was both the ambition to achieve this goal and the associated sense of responsibility that pushed us on. If we knew how to save thousands of lives with our central line checklist and associated CUSP program, we had a duty to share that knowledge.

With this goal in mind we recruited Chris Goeschel to come work with us in Baltimore. Her vision and determination literally made the Michigan success happen. I knew I would need that strength beside me if we planned to take on an entire country. Equipped with all our new skills and our ever-growing team of safety experts, we were ready to broadly implement the Michigan program.

Our next big project was in New Jersey. We rallied the troops, assembled all our new tools, and marched into the Garden State with high hopes and the best intentions. Two years later I found myself standing on stage in the uncomfortable position of telling a large crowd of well-intentioned New Jersey health care workers that we didn't know whether or not we had been successful in our attempt to reduce central line infections there.

# Chapter 7

At the end of our project in New Jersey, hundreds of hard-working, dedicated doctors, nurses, and administrators, as well as reporters from major media outlets in the state, had gathered for a press conference at the New Jersey Hospital Association Quality Institute in Princeton. I had been asked to give the keynote speech and everyone in the crowd, especially the reporters, were expecting me to report on how successful we had been. The hospital association had sent me graphs it had created suggesting a substantial reduction in infection rates. But I was far from convinced. I took the data and made an Excel spreadsheet in which hospitals were rows and the time periods in which they had to submit data were columns. I made each box with missing data red. The spreadsheet lit up like a stop sign—more than 60 percent of the data required was missing. As I stepped up to the mike, my heart felt like lead.

I know you tried hard, I know you wanted so much for this project to work. Yet I cannot tell from the data you submitted whether or not it has. I know some hospitals reduced these infections, but when more than 60 percent of the data from the

participating hospitals is missing, there is little I can scientifically conclude about the state as a whole, except that you have
a lot of missing data. I wish I could celebrate with you and tell
you all your patients are safer. I cannot. Some of your hospitals definitely did improve; but we do not know if overall the
whole state improved. Though it might appear as though it did,
the hospitals that submitted data before we implemented interventions are not the same as those that submitted data after
we implemented interventions. Therefore, it is impossible to
say conclusively that there was an overall reduction across the
state. You can ignore my interpretation and continue to believe
that we made all hospitals in the state safer for patients. Or you
can leave here knowing that we are capable of doing better,
that all the hospitals and clinicians in New Jersey are capable
of collecting good data and of truly reducing these infections
the way 103 ICUs in Michigan did. I am sure we can do better
and I know you want to. I am sure we can make New Jersey's
hospitals safer for patients like Josie King or anyone who walks
into their doors.

It was a hard speech to deliver. I knew that many in the state had
worked very hard and deserved better results, but what could I do?
I am a scientist and believe deeply that any conclusions about improvements in safety should be based on valid data. Unfortunately,
the data was incomplete and as such we could not make any real
conclusions. New Jersey is not unique; this is the norm for patient
safety and quality improvement efforts in this country. Data quality control is rarely if ever even considered. We believe we must set
higher standards before we can make any conclusions about patient
safety.

When the New Jersey Hospital Association (NJHA) first called and asked if we would bring our work to New Jersey they told us we would be working in partnership with other quality improvement experts. Eager to spread our program across the country, we arranged a meeting to discuss the project.

We met in the NJHA headquarters in Princeton. From the beginning it was clear we differed in how we thought the program should be run. We wanted to run it just like in Michigan, but they didn't want our model. They liked the central line checklist but they wanted to package it with what we thought was a cluttered hodgepodge of unrelated quality improvement programs and house these all inside their model—commonly known as "Plan Do Study Act" (PDSA) model. In PDSA researchers come up with a plan, try it out, observe the results, and then make it policy. PDSA is a twenty-five-year-old generic model that doesn't fit every scenario to which it is applied. And in this case our team did not think it fit well with what we wanted to accomplish.

What we primarily disagreed on was that the New Jersey team did not want to use standardized data collection tools or a centralized database or to conduct data quality control. Data was to be collected and used locally, by each hospital in whatever manner it saw fit. This program might be successful if we were only trying to make conclusions about what happened in one hospital in the state (though without data standards even that is suspect). However, it's a disaster if we wanted to try to make conclusions about what happened in a group of hospitals or the entire state.

It was a frustrating meeting. The Michigan undertaking was one of the most successful patient safety improvement projects ever conducted; and one of the keys to its success was valid centralized measurement. After listening to what they had to say, I gathered myself together and suggested we replicate what we did in Michigan; it was a practical yet scientifically sound solution. And it had a proven track record.

But the New Jersey group leaders told me that although they realized we had great success in Michigan, they had been doing patient safety work for a long time and preferred to use their model.

I tried to explain that we didn't use PDSA in Michigan, and that without good data collection we would never know if we actually improved safety. But it was clear the meeting was over. We had agreed to disagree and I left for Baltimore. I was disappointed, but in many ways I was not surprised. The checklist probably made sense to them; it's logical, it's easy to use, it's effective. I am sure they figured all they had to do was use the checklist and they would get the same results as Michigan. But we knew that the checklist doesn't work without both culture work and valid measurement.

Our team has learned from experience that reliable data collection is what separates mumbo jumbo from science, hope from reality. We viewed quality improvement as science—and scientific experiments demand robust and correct data. Specifically, each hospital had to use the same data collection tools, the same database, and the same data quality control methods to produce the same kind of data. If the data doesn't match between hospitals, it's like comparing apples and oranges. And apples and oranges would make it impossible for us to conclude that our checklist had reduced bloodstream infections across the state. If we let each hospital develop its own data collection process, we'd have the research equivalent of a fruit basket and much of it would be rotting, swooning with flies.

Another problem with local data collection is it's notoriously sloppy and incomplete. We had this problem in Michigan. In the early stages of the study we let each hospital be responsible for its own data collection. The results? We were missing almost 70 percent of the data we needed for our study. Once we centralized data collection and got hospitals to comply with the same standards, missing data dropped to 5 percent.

In addition, it is not efficient for individual hospitals to develop their own measures, data collection forms, and databases, and also analyze the data. Central data collection is more cost-effective and takes less time.

It is not surprising that our proposed methods met resistance. The rigorous data collection we were proposing was novel. Few in the patient safety and quality improvement world asked for accurate, high-quality data in patient safety or quality improvement work. In fact, there are barely any published articles written on data quality in quality improvement. Essentially we were coming at them with something they hadn't seen before. Therefore it was easy to dismiss, especially since it was potentially time intensive.

At my second meeting with the New Jersey team I tried to better understand their view. They have worked on quality improvement and patient safety a great deal and are experienced with implementing interventions, though less experienced with evaluating them. I explained that I was not sure exactly why our programs had been so successful at Hopkins and Michigan. All I could tell for sure was that the checklist, cultural changes, and collecting data worked and they worked as a unit—when you do all three, you get results; when people try to tear them apart, the whole thing fails.

But the New Jersey team was reluctant to give any ground. They said they were comfortable with their model and had been using it for some time. It was obvious they did not see rigorous measurement as critical; more specifically, that there was really no place for it

within their model. Doubtful of the success of the project, I decided
not to participate.

I felt I was right to stick to my principles, to what I did in Michigan, to making patient safety a science. But I had my doubts. What
we were doing was still experimental. It might have worked at Hopkins and in Michigan, but that was no guarantee it would work everywhere. I knew it was not a perfect model and that we were always
learning. Perhaps the New Jersey undertaking would be another opportunity for our work to grow stronger. As I was walking out of the
building a nurse from one of the hospitals came up to me and said,
"We are so excited to learn from you. We have patients dying needlessly all the time. The idea that your project will happen here has
brought us energy to improve."

This chance encounter softened the hard exterior that had been
created by those difficult meetings. Perhaps I was letting my ego get
in the way. Maybe I didn't have all the answers. Maybe we could
learn from the New Jersey team's approach to patient safety.

I went back into the room and sat down with the sole desire of
finding some kind of compromise. The mood was still a bit awkward
given our different points of view. Yet I kept reminding myself that
we were both committed to patient safety and neither of us wanted
to walk away from this opportunity. After much maneuvering, and
some good will and effort from the New Jersey team members, we
managed to find a middle ground. They agreed to include the culture component of CUSP, and I gave in on the measurement issue.
In my heart and mind I was still unsure about our chances for reducing central line infections across the state, but I owed it to patients in
New Jersey to give it a try.

When we finished our work, the New Jersey team saw it as a
great success—approximately forty hospitals in the state had ICU

teams participating, and all were fully engaged in the program. The final meeting was held with great excitement and fanfare. Clinicians, hospital leaders, members of the boards of trustees, and the press were invited to celebrate the reduction of central line infections statewide. There were discussions about coordinating press conferences, rewarding teams, and briefing boards of trustees.

But the data did not support this conclusion. It is true that a couple of hospitals reduced their rates substantially (and were cited as examples) but the harsh reality was that for most hospitals, we had no idea whether they reduced their infections.

The New Jersey team was not trying to deceive anyone. All of us wanted desperately to improve safety. They were following the traditional methods of quality improvement and they truly believed they had lowered the rates of infections in the state. Yet few people in patient safety are trained in research methods and therefore cannot be expected to apply research standards to quality improvement.

The message of the state's success got sent to reporters, who were invited to a press conference where the news would be announced publicly. It was there that I gave my fated speech telling all gathered that they I was unsure whether infections rates were reduced in the state as a whole.

It was a terrible moral dilemma. Everyone obviously expected me to say the initiative had worked. The people had put a lot of effort into the program and were engaged and excited. Truthfully, New Jersey did have some success with the program. Teams across the state implemented the checklist, used CUSP and daily goals, improved culture, and learned from mistakes. Many of the hospitals described it as a transformative experience and I suspect it was. Doctors and nurses were now making rounds together, communicating better, and learning from mistakes. And in fact, several hospitals did collect accurate data and made dramatic reductions in infections rates.

Our work needed this passion and enthusiasm. The last thing I wanted to do was discourage future efforts. Yet as important as it is to have clinicians engaged in improving quality, patients aren't safer without valid results. If I agreed with this misleading conclusion, patients would continue to suffer harm. Not only that but I felt I would be committing scientific misconduct. I would be going against everything I held sacred. Linking safety work with science is one of the core missions of my work. I knew there was no way I could go on stage and talk against all I had been fighting for all these years, against what I believed in my heart.

I remembered a national quality improvement meeting I attended a few years back. A "researcher" was presenting the results of the efforts of over twenty hospitals to reduce pneumonia rates. She heralded the project as a stunning success, yet the data she was using was junk. Missing data exceeded available data and different hospitals submitted data in different time periods. When a physician in the audience challenged her, citing the poor data and biased study design, the presenter said, "This data is for quality improvement, not research." As if labeling something as quality improvement gives you a free pass for making inaccurate conclusions. When I heard that, my stomach churned and I vowed never to make that kind of statement or take that approach in my own work. I would instead do whatever it took to bring more robust research methods to quality improvement and patient safety; the public deserves to have accurate data.

Shortly after we started the New Jersey project we had a similar disappointment. Only this time I terminated the contract early in the project. The Maryland Hospital Association and a well-known quality improvement organization joined forces and created the

Maryland Patient Safety Center (MPSC)—an organization similar to the Keystone Center in Michigan. The MPSC called and told us they wanted to do our project. But like the team in New Jersey, the MPSC didn't want to follow the Michigan model. They wanted to use local, nonstandardized methods for data collection and add a large number of additional interventions to the project that I felt would distract teams.

I respected their desire to improve patient safety and was honored that they wanted our team to be a part of that effort. But it seemed like they had a different approach and different ideas. What bothered me most was they did not want to put resources toward supporting valid centralized data collection. I regretted having agreed to run the New Jersey program without this essential component and was not willing to make the same mistake again. So I contacted the head of the center and politely announced that we could not participate in the project. This was especially disappointing for me because Maryland is my home state and I care deeply about improving the patient safety there.

These back-to-back disappointments had really taken the wind out of our sails. We were trying to develop more robust methods in quality improvement yet the majority of the field had been doing it the same way for many years and was reluctant to change. We wanted to bridge the gap between the sincere efforts of these quality improvement groups and the hard science that my fellow physicians and researchers demanded so they could be sure that quality improvement efforts actually improve patient outcomes. It was a tough balancing act, but I was determined to get these two groups together.

After these experiences what our team needed was some really good news, and it came via Rhode Island congressman Patrick

Kennedy. Kennedy invited me to his office in Washington, D.C., to discuss health reform. I have to admit I had great expectations before I even entered his office. The Kennedy family had always been champions of the people, of important causes—battling for civil rights, fighting organized crime, and creating the Special Olympics. Perhaps I was being unrealistic, but I truly believed Representative Kennedy would understand our work and embrace and support it in its entirety. While waiting in his office I studied the picture of Patrick's uncles Bobby and John Kennedy alongside the pictures of his father, Ted. By the time the congressman entered the room, my hopes were high; I was ready to make Rhode Island the next Michigan.

It was a pleasant meeting. Kennedy asked me pointed questions about our work at Hopkins and Michigan and I told him I was sure we could do the same in Rhode Island. I could tell he liked the idea and he said that he would look into it.

It was an enjoyable meeting. We got along well. He even invited me to a party at the Kennedy Compound on Cape Cod for Ted Kennedy and Hillary Clinton. I thanked him, but I was scheduled to be in the ICU and could not attend. However, I told him my mother lived on Cape Cod and would love to go. He sent my mom two tickets and she invited Paul Buckley, the man she would later marry. This was their first date and they had a great time. The Kennedys are revered, especially on Cape Cod, and my mom was excited just to see the compound and meet Ted and Hillary.

However, in spite of his warmth and congeniality, I was not sure whether Congressman Kennedy was truly interested in our work or if I was only a checkmark on his long list of possible projects. I was hopeful, but I wasn't expecting to hear from him all that quickly. Happily, I was wrong.

Within a week I got a call from Laura Adams, the CEO of the Rhode Island Quality Institute, a not-for-profit organization that was in charge of improving quality of health care in Rhode Island. I had known Laura for years; she was a tireless worker and had done great things for quality improvement. She understood the science and believed in the importance of accurate data. She had received a grant to improve quality of care in her state and wanted to use some of that money to implement our program. And, most important, Laura wanted to do the whole shebang: the checklist, the culture work, and centralized data collection. It was music to my ears. She trusted our methods and was wise enough to recognize that the public would and should demand robust data.

However, to use a Kennedy metaphor, it wasn't all smooth sailing. Rhode Island had its own set of challenges. What is patient safety work if you don't have a little resistance? Yet in this case it wasn't resistance, it was overenthusiasm.

In the past, we struggled to get infectious disease experts on board with our program. In Rhode Island, however, the infectious disease teams were so eager and anxious to participate they wanted to practically run the show. However, as we learned at Hopkins and in Michigan, nurses and ICU doctors have to own this problem, not infectious disease practitioners. If Rhode Island's infectious disease teams ran this program, nothing would likely change. The solution to these infections must lie with the caregivers at the bedside, not with infectious disease practitioners. At Hopkins and in Michigan, we partnered with infection control experts and used their expertise to help educate staff and monitor infections. But we made the bedside doctors and nurses in the ICU accountable.

In the beginning, infection control experts often dominated the conference calls. It was tough going for a while. But we trudged forward, convinced that once we got the cultural changes of CUSP in place everyone would remember that the patient was the focus not turf battles. We told stories of actual errors and how patients had paid for these mistakes—often with their lives. Eventually, people started to come around, thanks, in great part, to some visionary leadership from a few key Rhode Island players—specifically Vera DePalo, a gregarious and passionate ICU physician, and Leonard Mermel, an infectious disease physician who is a world leader in infection control. These two brilliant doctors were able to melt the tensions, unite the community, and get the work done. They recognized that both infection control and ICU clinicians needed to be engaged, but ICU clinicians needed to be accountable.

Thanks to their efforts, infection control experts joined the ICU CUSP teams and everyone started working together toward the common goal. It was clearly a testimony to the power of our model in general and CUSP in particular. With all the wheels of our program turning at once—checklist, culture, and measurement—Rhode Island, predictably, had virtually the same results as Michigan.

In spite of our success in Rhode Island, we were still struggling to spread our central line infection program across the United States. However, in the midst of this struggle, we received some unexpected interest from across the Atlantic. At an international conference in Barcelona, a brilliant and prominent ICU physician named Mercedes Palomar asked Chris about our work. By the end of the day, Mercedes had invited Chris and me to visit Spain to see if there was a chance we could start some of this work in her country.

A month later, we were talking to Spanish health care officials about implementing the program across the country. We told them that we believed culture would be the biggest barrier. Moving from the ICU to the operating room, or from one U.S. state to another, was one thing, but crossing the Atlantic was a big shift. The checklist and its associated technical components were easily translated. Yet, we believed our culture work would need to be tailored to fit Spain's unique culture—specifically, the way Spanish clinicians worked together. However, we reassured the minister that we were confident we could overcome these obstacles. Since Mercedes had been working for years to monitor infection rates in the ICU she proved to be an excellent colleague for this work. She had already developed a good system for measuring rates of infection, which we learned were quite high.

We agreed to pilot test the project in nine ICUs. As expected, the clinicians in each ICU put more emphasis on the checklist than they did on the culture work. The pilot program stalled and Mercedes asked for input. When we met to discuss the problem, she said that she had focused heavily on the checklist and measurement but neglected the culture work because she knew that it would be challenging and messy.

It was clear that the way medical teams interacted in Spain was very different from how it worked in the United States. The dynamic between doctors and nurses in Spain was even more hierarchical. Nurses rarely spoke up and often did not participate in rounds. There was no perceived need for them to participate. They were never invited to physician conferences, rarely consulted about patients, and, in general, were treated like second-class citizens.

Mercedes recognized that this needed to change. I asked her if we could invite nurses to the next national critical care conference as a way to put doctors and nurses on equal footing. She said she thought it was an excellent idea. The conference was a huge success and helped begin to break down long-standing walls. I gave the keynote speech, calling for the clinicians to reduce these infections and explaining that this would require much greater teamwork than they had done in the past. Energy was high—doctors, nurses, and health ministers became aligned toward the common goal, eliminating infections. The politics changed from one of exclusion to one of inclusion. In a small way, culture began gradually changing in these ICUs.

With this improved culture and an increased focus on CUSP, we had tremendous success reducing infection rate. We are currently implementing the program nationwide.

Word got out about our work in Spain and other countries started to express interest. The World Health Organization's Patient Safety Program was already supporting our work in Spain so we asked them to help us implement the program across Europe and the world. We used the same strategy that worked in Spain. First garner interest from each nation's health minister—who would serve a similar role as the Michigan Hospital Association did in Michigan. Then test a pilot program in a small group of hospitals to identify what part of the program worked and what part needed to be modified. This pilot test (and the program itself) would be led by an ICU leader from within the country.

Not long after we started working in Spain, we were invited to the United Kingdom to talk about instituting the program there. Amazingly, we learned that the U.K. monitors several hundred performance measures yet does not routinely measure central line infection rates. It was clear that we could not determine if the U.K. had a problem with central line infections until we measured them. If we found a problem then we could talk about taking action to lower them. The National Patient Safety Agency (NPSA) held a planning meeting with leaders in critical care and microbiology where we discussed the possibility of running a pilot study to measure the rates. The meeting opened with many of the physicians acting defensively. Several of the doctors said that central line infections were not a problem in the United Kingdom. They said they had already implemented interventions to reduce central line infections and were not enthusiastic about repeating work they thought they had already done. It was true that many hospitals in the U.K. had implemented our central line checklist, but none had implemented culture change or measured results. Unfortunately, this led doctors to believe there wasn't a problem.

We told them we were not challenging their expertise, we simply wanted to measure the rates and let the data guide us. If we found high infection rates we could then talk about ways to lower the rates. The U.K. doctors clearly saw the logic in this approach and agreed to a pilot study that would measure the rates of these infections in eighteen ICUs in the northeast region of England.

We worked with British leaders in ICU care and microbiology to develop definitions for infection and how we would collect the data. Chris and I consulted regularly, sharing tools and strategies, visiting hospitals, and talking to frontline caregivers and senior leaders. We shared all that we had learned from the Michigan project and all that we had learned since, and we watched them make it their own. The results were striking: the infection rates in some of the hospitals were as high or higher than the rates in Michigan before our program.

Everyone now understood that perceptions and data often don't agree. As a result, our program gained substantial momentum. Some of the country's senior anesthesiologists became true CUSP champions. We had support from the United Kingdom's minister of health, who at the time we began was Lord Ara Darzi; and also had support from Sir Liam Donaldson, who is both the chief medical officer for England, and the U.K.'s chief medical adviser to the World Health Organization (WHO). In addition we had support from Dr. Julian Bion, a prominent critical care physician in the U.K.

Thanks to our success, we are now running a pilot program to lower central line infection rates in those eighteen ICUs. If this is successful (and we are sure it will be) we will likely spread the program across the U.K.

The work in the U.K. and Spain continues to gain momentum. The energy and success surrounding those projects have inspired us to keep expanding. In fact we have recently started working with Peru, using the same model—engaging the minister of health and physician leaders, pilot testing in a sample of hospitals, and making a plan to spread it throughout the country. Thanks to support from WHO, we will continue to take our work around the globe.

As exciting as all this is, it only further highlights the lack of interest back home. It isn't from lack of publicity. After the *New England Journal of Medicine* published our Michigan work, the scientific community sat up and took notice. We were one of the first, if not the first, to develop a large-scale solution to hospital error and quality of care that was backed with valid scientific data. Leading researchers in the field cited our work as one of the most important studies in the last decade. Others commented that this intervention could save more lives than virtually any other medical therapy of the last quarter century.

Stories of our success appeared in the *Wall Street Journal*, the *New York Times*, and *The New Yorker*, as well as countless other magazine and newspapers. I was named one of *Time* magazine's one hundred most influential people in 2008 and was one of twenty-five people nationally to receive the coveted MacArthur Fellowship. This was the validation we needed. We have proven, to ourselves and to the world, that we can make hospitals and patients safer, not only at Johns Hopkins but in Michigan and Rhode Island and in Europe. We have shown that using a scientific approach to patient safety and quality improvement—an approach that includes evidence-based practices, substantive culture change, and good measurement—will make hospitals safer. We have introduced a new paradigm. Patient safety and quality improvement have officially won their place at the table of science. Hospitals and clinicians now demand robust data before making conclusions about quality and safety: a new science is emerging.

Still, in spite of all this success, states were not calling. We knew one of the main reasons was money. States didn't have the funding they needed to implement the program, nor did we. We had a little money from the U.S. government; but aside from that, we were going it alone. If this program were a drug or a device we would have had enormous support from government and industry. If we had found the cure to AIDS or cancer, the world would be beating a path to our door with checks in hand. But safety and quality control are hard to quantify. This kind of work is often invisible. Two and a half million people died from hospital-acquired bloodstream infections in the United States over the last twenty-five years, yet the entire budget that year for the Agency for Healthcare Research and Quality was only $300 million.

One of the main reasons for this lack of funding is that patient safety is largely invisible. Most errors go undetected and unidentified. When a patient in the ICU contracts a bloodstream infection from a central line and dies, the family is not told that he died from a preventable infection. Instead, loved ones are told the death was due to "complications related to his illness and surgery." In some cases, the man may have died whether or not he got a bloodstream infection, but often it's the infection that kills. Who can blame hospitals for not broadcasting this fact? It's bad for business and also can attract expensive lawsuits. But if we don't talk about it, it will never get fixed. Our goal is to get this menace out in the open. The public needs to know the scope of the problem, that it is endemic throughout health care, and that the solution lies in wiping out these infections, not attacking the hospitals and doctors. These infections are not the only risk to patients; there are many others. Yet the medical community has a very poor track record of solving patient safety problems. I believe we need to learn how to work together to really lick this problem and in doing so, build capacity to address many of the other ills that befall health care. These infections could be the polio campaign of the twenty-first century and we need government support to make it happen.

Understandably, safety research in general is harder to sell than a typical drug trial. Pills and devices that improve outcomes and save lives are easy to understand. You're sick, you take a new pill, you get better—everyone gets it, everyone is on board. The pill is picked up by manufacturers, produced, and marketed. Costs come down and quality goes up. Hospitals everywhere adopt its use. The business model and incentives are aligned, assuming the drug or device actually works.

Safety research, however, looks for ways to prevent harm—like avoiding central line infections or wrong-site surgeries. When safety programs are successful, nothing happens. A nonevent is much harder to conceptualize than a drug, and it is often invisible. Policy makers are reluctant to throw money at anything unless they can point to concrete outcomes. And we desperately needed money to continue working. Our research team was living off of grants and

contracts; without financial support our team would need to disband. If something didn't break soon, I was afraid we would never
achieve our dream of ending central line infections across the United
States.

And then, like magic, Barack Obama and health care reform
appeared on the horizon, and suddenly we saw a possible way to get
the funding support we so desperately needed. As soon as it became
apparent that the Democrats were going to return to power, the
glacier surrounding funding for patient safety programs started to
thaw. All the big players in Congress knew health care reform was
going to be a significant agenda item. And everyone wanted to be
well positioned on the issue long before inauguration day. The great
press we received for our work in Michigan and the MacArthur
grant had put us on the radar screen, and calls from senators and
congresspeople started trickling in. And so I entered the next phase
of my patient safety career—Beltway politics.

# Chapter 8

═══

Politicians loved the central line checklist. It was simple to explain and easy to implement, it had proven results, and, most important, it didn't cost a lot of money. For senators and congresspeople looking for health care reform that could translate easily into crisp, meaty sound bites—the checklist was made to order.

I was okay with this fascination with the checklist. If it got us in the door, so be it. Once I was "inside," I'd push the culture change and measurement aspects of our work, but for now, the checklist was our passkey.

One of the first politicians to contact my office was Democratic senator Sherrod Brown from Ohio. One of his staffers called me and asked if I might be willing to come down to Washington for a fifteen-minute meeting to talk about reducing bloodstream infections; fifteen minutes is all you get when you meet with a top-ranking U.S. official.

My goal was to build relationships and gain support for our work from these powerful leaders. We needed to expand our program nationally and we needed someone with large-scale influence to help make that happen. Senators had that kind of influence. We arrived at Senator Brown's office in the Russell Senate Office Building and were ushered into a wood-paneled conference room. His staffers, as well as staffers for Senators Edward Kennedy and Barbara Mikulski, were waiting for him. We talked while Brown's assistant kept us abreast of his estimated arrival time.

When Senator Brown finally arrived, I immediately liked him. He had brown wavy hair that reminded me of my father's, neither overly groomed nor unkempt. The connection gave me automatic trust. With his gruff voice and matter-of-fact questions, he continued to impress me as an honest representative of the people. In fact Senator Brown has a reputation for looking out for the common man. I was sure he would be interested to know what our checklist could do for his state.

I gave him a quick overview of our work reducing bloodstream infections at Hopkins and in Michigan. He seemed to be very interested in what I had to say, in terms of both national health care policy and the impact bloodstream infections might be having on patients in Ohio. Just as I had expected, once Brown learned about the risk of these infections and our success in eliminating them, he wanted to find a way to implement this program in his state. It was inspiring to see this powerful and influential leader get excited about our work. After our meeting, he actually got on the phone with the Ohio Hospital Association and asked, point-blank, "Why aren't we doing Peter's checklist?"

Much to my surprise, my fifteen minutes with Senator Brown turned into thirty minutes and then an hour. The senator's assistant kept informing him that he had other obligations but he waved her off saying he needed to hear what we were saying and that it was important. I sensed that he knew health reform would be big with the new president, who was likely to be a Democrat. As a member of the powerful Senate Committee on Health, Education, Labor and Pensions (HELP), which was a major player in health reform, Senator Brown needed to be well informed on the issues so he could lead health reform efforts. The senator told me there was a growing group of senators, Democrats and Republicans alike, who were interested in improving the quality of health care. He wanted to introduce them to our program.

In the end we spent an hour and a half together—an eternity for a senator. I also got a sample of the awesome power these senators wield. Shortly after our meeting, I received a shocked and confused call from the director of the Ohio Hospital Association responding to Senator Brown's earlier call. "Peter," she said, "we would love to use your program but we have to find out how to pay for it. We are working to obtain financial support to do this, yet without some funding we can't do it."

Hospital associations have the same problem as the rest of us in getting support for this kind of work—hospitals usually don't reap the bulk of the financial rewards for these efforts, health insurers do. And since multiple insurers compete with each other, individual companies are reluctant to pay because the benefits of their investments are shared with their competitors. That left only one possible source of revenue, the federal government. Since these projects produced a public good—saving lives and money—it only made sense that they be financed with public money. (For example, Michigan earned back roughly two hundred dollars in savings for every dollar invested in our grant.) But I knew government officials were more likely to support biomedical research (drugs and devices) than safety research. That was why it was essential that I impress upon these powerful legislators that safety research was just as important to support.

Senator Ted Kennedy also invited me to come and talk about our work. Recently named chairman of the Senate HELP Committee, he also needed to be well educated on health care reform. Kennedy was too sick at the time to meet with me, so I met with his staffer Dr. Kavita Patel. According to her, when Kennedy heard about our work in Michigan he said it had to go national.

Kavita said they liked my work because while hundreds of health care reformers use aviation analogies and talk about improving quality, very few have done it. Even those who have done it have no data to support their claims. "I like this story because it's good science and it works. It saves lives and money. You are talking about change at a policy level but you're doing it on the ground. You also have data I believe in and nobody else has had that. So we're comfortable supporting it because we believe it works," she said.

It was music to my ears. We were talking scientist to scientist and were both on the same page. These alliances clearly demonstrated the credibility of our work. And it provided further support to me about the wisdom of our model. Without data—and justifiably so—we wouldn't be advising Congress.

But all of these encounters also came with a dose of anxiety for me. It's one thing to fail at Hopkins or in a state. It's entirely different and rather intimidating to imagine failure on the national stage, with hospital administrators and clinical teams across the country relying on our leadership. The mantle of responsibility is even heavier when senators and congresspeople trust your message and embrace your recommendations. And failure could easily happen. Science is messy; there is always a risk that the experiment could go wrong.

Maryland senator Barbara Mikulski also was eager to speak with me. A member of the Senate HELP Committee, she had been named by Kennedy to lead the Senate's hearings on improving health care quality. And like her fellow senators, she wanted to get her facts straight. But she had additional reason to be interested in my work. Hopkins is one of the biggest employers in Maryland and Mikulski is a huge supporter. When she learned that a physician from Hopkins was leading an important cause for health care reform she was behind us 100 percent.

Senator Mikulski, like Senator Brown, is also a champion of the people. A native of Highlandtown, a classic blue-collar neighborhood in East Baltimore, Senator Mikulski had made a career out of taking issues away from bureaucrats and putting them where they belong—with the citizens. A powerhouse of energy and enthusiasm condensed into a four foot, eleven-inch frame, she has a sweet smile, a good heart, and fierce determinism. I knew that if Mikulski believed in an idea she could be a great ally.

After years of feeling as though we were fighting this battle alone, it was empowering to finally have interest and support from people we knew could really make a difference. Our message was clear. Patient safety is science, and like all research, it must have ample federal funding. Yet patient safety research is grossly underfunded. If we can increase its budget substantially, we will save lives and money almost immediately.

As exciting and inspiring as it was to get the ear of powerful senators, the most significant call I received came from Dr. Stephen Cha, health care adviser to Congressman Henry Waxman of California. Representative Waxman, at the time, chaired the Committee on Oversight and Government Reform. After hearing about the number of people dying from hospital-acquired infections, Waxman commissioned a report from the Government Accountability Office (GAO) that examined federal efforts to reduce hospital-acquired infections. The report was blunt and factual. Its conclusion: the federal efforts to reduce health care–acquired infections have been fragmented and for the most part inadequate. There is little or no coordination among federal agencies to fight these infections and a gross lack of accountability. This must change.

Waxman learned about our success fighting central line infections in Michigan and wanted me to come to Washington and testify about what we did in Michigan and how it could act as a national model. I was honored he'd asked me to participate, but I was also uneasy. Casual conversations with senators and their staff were one thing, but testifying before Congress was another. I believed the government could do much more to address this important issue. But how could I make this message clear "on record" without insulting government officials who could be great allies in this struggle? It would be a delicate balance for someone who was new to all this.

Chris and several members of Hopkins' government relations team accompanied me on the train from Baltimore. We walked in the chilly winter air from Union Station to the Rayburn House Office Building where the hearing was scheduled to take place. Scores of people were lined up outside waiting to enter. After passing though the metal detector, I was taken into a holding room for speakers. As always, I planned to make the patient the focus of my testimony. I planned to outline a strategy to improve patient safety, and I would stress that it would take the efforts of many to achieve this goal. Some of my message would question current government efforts and therefore make some people uncomfortable. However, you can't make change without challenging status quo, and we needed change desperately.

There were a number of people presenting along with me, but by far the one who impressed me the most was Edward Lawton, a retired air force officer who had been confined to a wheelchair because of a infection from so-called superbug methicillin-resistant Staphylococcus aureus (MRSA). Lawton had orthopedic surgery for a knee replacement that became infected with MRSA. This infection, though largely preventable, is notoriously difficult to clear. Like many other patients with MRSA infections in their bones, Lawton underwent multiple and expensive surgeries, with long hospital stays, that ultimately resulted in him being confined to a wheelchair—probably costing over a million dollars and years of pain and suffering. His story was moving. To me, Lawton was the Josie King of that hearing; he grounded me and made these discussions real. Like Josie, Lawton put the focus on the patient where it belongs and made sure that message was not lost or diluted by policy talk. Errors kill and harm real people.

In fact, I was so moved listening to Lawton's story, I decided to open my talk with a reference to him. "What happened to Mr. Lawton should never happen again. We can prevent most health care–acquired infections and we need to ensure we do; it will not be easy, it will take viewing patient safety as a science, it will take more collaboration than we have had in the past, and it will take your leadership. Yet we can do it."

I followed that extemporaneous introduction with a detailed explanation of our work. I talked about the wonders of medical research and how it is tragic that there is no national program that ensures patients receive the new life-saving treatments that are funded with taxpayer dollars through the NIH. I noted the lack of government support, clear goals, and quantifiable, explicit strategies among federal agencies and others to reduce infections. I presented the results of what we had done in Michigan and asked for federal leadership to spread it to all the states. I assured everyone in that

room that if given the chance, if provided with the necessary support, we could eliminate bloodstream infections across the country;
we could make hospitals safer so what happened to Mr. Lawton
would not happen again.

I crammed all of this into a three-minute speech. I was not used
to giving such short talks and it forced me to hone my message,
to find the right balance between stories and facts, and to present
concrete recommendations. I thanked them for their time and took
my seat. It seemed to be well received; I was hopeful it would lead
to action.

Shortly after the hearing, Stephen Cha called to tell me Representative Waxman could not believe that my checklist was not used
nationally and that they were going to do something about that.
Although I was new to politics, I was beginning to understand if you
get the message into the right ear at the right time, it can really make
a big difference.

It wasn't long before I got a second call from Stephen telling
me that they planned to survey all the states to see what they were
doing to fight bloodstream infections. I was ecstatic that someone
was finally listening to me, that someone was finally taking action.
However, when Stephen sent me the survey, it wasn't exactly what
I had in mind. The survey asked state hospital associations point-
blank whether the hospitals in their state were using the "Pronovost
checklist" to prevent bloodstream infections. While I liked the idea
of evaluating what each state was doing, I thought patient safety had
for too long focused on efforts rather than results.

"Stephen," I said, "I don't care if they say they are using my
checklist. People like Sorrel and Lawton don't care, either. What
I need to know is what the infection rates are in these hospitals. If
they are high, we need to know what they are doing about them."

Stephen clearly understood my dilemma. It wasn't about the checklist; it was about the patient. Our work at Hopkins proved that you can give clinicians a checklist, but if it's not used properly, if nurses do not question physicians, if culture does not improve, the infection rates won't go down. And the only way to know that the checklist is being used correctly is to measure results.

As a result of my request, Waxman amended the survey to ask whether the states measured bloodstream infection rates and what those rates were. It was amazing. After struggling for so long, feeling isolated in our work, we finally had found a powerful ally who understood our vision. And what a powerful ally he turned out to be. When a hospital association receives a survey from the chairman of the Committee on Oversight and Government Reform, it gets attention.

All fifty states promptly responded to the survey, and all reported that their institutions were using the "Pronovost checklist," as well as a number of other programs, to reduce infections. This was not surprising. The Michigan study received a lot of acclaim and attention. The IHI had launched a national campaign, part of which was to use the checklist to reduce central line infections. Most states and thousand of hospitals participated. Yet the measurement of infections was generally not part of these programs and as such, only eleven state hospital associations reported monitoring infection rates and no state had come even close to getting rates as low as Michigan's. (To be fair, many hospital associations were not charged with measuring infections; their state health departments were. And even if they wanted to, many lacked resources to monitor these infections.)

We also got another response, one of frustration and anger. My colleagues at the Michigan Hospital Association called me and said they had received calls from other state hospital associations complaining that they didn't like the way we were shining this congressional spotlight on their infection rates. My office was also inundated with similar calls. Their representatives complained that Michigan had set an unrealistic example by nearly eliminating bloodstream infections, and that it wasn't possible across the nation. Hospital associations believed they were working hard on the problem, even if they did not have results. My response to each hospital association was simple. I told them that I understood their concerns but that you can't fight infections if you don't know the extent of the problem; and similarly, you can't judge the success of your efforts unless you measure results. I said that we wouldn't promote our program unless we felt it could have the same results in other states that it had in Michigan. I concluded by suggesting that their hospitals should start monitoring their infection rates so they could ensure that their citizens were not needlessly being harmed. Health care needs to be held accountable.

Despite this blowback, we had at least gotten everyone's attention. Moreover, nearly all agreed that we should monitor and reduce infections; we just needed to find the resources to do so. Washington had flexed its muscles and now states had to take action, whether they wanted to or not. Now all we needed was money, and that was on its way.

The Waxman survey created a new wave of interest in our work and my phone was ringing off the hook with people who wanted to know more about our program. Many of the calls I received were from lawyers and businesspeople offering to help me profit from my work. They believed the work we were doing had significant value and should be converted into a for-profit company. I was torn about this. We were desperately in need of funding, but I was uneasy about creating a for-profit company. While I knew the discipline of market competition would likely lead to more effective and efficient safety programs, I also knew that safety was fragile. I had the bully pulpit in part because we produced results, but also because our program was purely patient focused: there were no hidden agendas or conflicts of interest. I sincerely believed that it would be much harder to get states on board if we were a for-profit company. I decided this work, ultimately, needs to be in the public space. I discussed this issue with my wife, Chris, Ed Miller, and Bill Brody, then president of Johns Hopkins University, and all agreed.

Still I needed capital to do the work. While I was optimistic that we would receive federal money to support our work, either as part of health reform or grants, I knew that would not happen quickly. We needed capital now.

One day when I was reviewing a list of calls that had come in I saw Herbert Sandler's name. He and his wife, Marion, once owned Golden West Financial and sold it to Wachovia at the peak of the real estate boom. They created the Sandler Foundation, one of the wealthiest foundations in the country, and donated large sums of money to medical research. On my drive home from work, I returned his call and he seemed to be very excited to hear about our work. Right after he hung up with me, Herb called Bill Brody to check up on me and make sure I was the right guy to be talking to about this move. Bill strongly recommended both me and my work to Sandler.

The next morning at seven a.m., while working on a research paper with a colleague, I got a call from Bill on my cell phone. Bill told me that Hopkins had been trying to get support from Sandler's foundation for years with no luck. Bill wanted to make sure I realized what a great opportunity this was.

Herb and I had several more calls. He wanted me to produce a formal proposal for an institute of patient safety housed on a medical school campus that would support our bloodstream infection work and other safety initiatives. Realizing the size of his foundation, I decided not to hold back. I drafted a proposal for $10 million a year for ten years. If I was really going to start an institute and have a big impact, I knew I would need this kind of money.

I was invited to visit Herb and Marion in San Francisco. I had dinner with the Sandlers and their lawyer shortly after my plane touched down. They peppered me with questions. At eight the next morning the inquisition started again. They wanted to know about my goals, my strategy, my vision, and me. I left exhausted and unnerved; it was hard to tell if they were truly interested in backing our work. After several more telephone calls about building a safety institute, I was invited to California for another in-person meeting. This one started as soon as I arrived in the San Francisco Airport. We discussed my business plan for creating a safety institute to coordinate and fund safety research. We went through each item and the budget in exquisite detail. After two hours, Herb smiled. He said, "The dance is over. We decided to fund you. Now we are a team, working together to realize your vision. And we can help you realize it."

I left excited. A couple of weeks later, Herb arranged another visit and gave his offer a condition. The majority of the Sandlers' philanthropy had traditionally been focused on the University of California, San Francisco (UCSF) and Herb wanted us to create the institute there.

My wife, Marlene, and I explored the possibility of moving to San Francisco. On one of the visits, Herb had arranged a meeting with other leaders in philanthropy and health care around San Francisco. It was impressive. The heads of the Google Foundation, the Gordon and Betty Moore Foundation, the California HealthCare Foundation, and the Henry J. Kaiser Family Foundation all seemed interested and they tried to lure me to UCSF. They had money and were looking for leadership with vision. Herb believed I filled that void. The potential to change health care with the help of the substantial financial and IT resources available in the Bay Area was real and very attractive.

Yet, there were a lot of problems with this move. For one, San Francisco was very expensive compared to Baltimore. Second, though UCSF is a great institution, I had built a team of safety researchers at Hopkins that was hard to match. I had colleagues in the Hopkins schools of public health and medicine that were indispensable. It would likely take me years to create such a team in California. Similarly, my wife had recently moved back to Hopkins and her career was exploding. Essentially, it was a big risk for my wife and me to take, based on one philanthropist's donation. That being said, I couldn't just walk away from the Sandlers' support; the program and patients desperately needed it. The reality was we had a proven system for making patients safer and no money to put it into action. Then another miracle happened.

A donor who wanted to remain anonymous heard me talk about safety. He also read the *New Yorker* article written about me and called to arrange a meeting. When we met, it was clear he liked what he heard. I was unsure whether I should mention the Sandler Foundation. I did not have a firm agreement with the Sandlers, yet I felt I needed to be honest about the their interest. So I told the donor about the Sandlers and said I would tell the Sandlers about the donor's interest. The donor, like the Sandlers, was truly supportive of the work and did not care if the program was branded in his name.

He wanted to save lives. He said he would anonymously donate $1.2 million if the Sandlers would match it.

I knew that $2.4 million would go a long way in helping reduce infection rates across the nation. Granted it wasn't the $100 million I had discussed with Herb for a UCSF-based institute, but perhaps we could put that idea on the back burner for now. Reducing blood-stream infections was the goal and this was clearly a worthwhile compromise.

Marlene and I arranged to have lunch with Herb and Marion at the Oregon Grille near our house. I had asked the trustee to put his offer in writing and brought a copy of that letter with me. It had now been six months that we had been negotiating with the Sandlers and I had little to show for it save higher cell phone bills and frequent flier miles. It was the first time Marlene had met the Sandlers. They got along well and talked at length about the institute. I kept rela-tively quiet. I had a lot on my mind. My wife and I were still uncer-tain about moving to San Francisco. Yet I knew that without a quick infusion of cash, I would have to disband my team and dream. I had a letter in my pocket that, if matched by the Sandlers, would solve these two problems. I could only hope that they would agree. After lunch, the waiter cleared the plates and brought coffee. I pulled out the letter and handed it across the table.

I said, "I have an offer for $1.2 million for this work, on the con-dition that you put in the same. This would allow you to double your investment. It would be a shame to lose this money. We can finalize whether we are moving to San Francisco at a later date. But this will at least let us get started hiring people and getting states on board. Many have called me to express interest."

Herb was known for being practical when it came to money and I was sure he would not want to throw away an opportunity to double his donation. He took the letter, read it, and said he would draw up papers the next day.

At that point, we only had one hurdle standing between our team and its dream to wipe out bloodstream infections across the country—and it wasn't a small one. About a year after we published our landmark Michigan study in the *New England Journal of Medicine*, an anonymous complaint regarding our study was filed at the Office for Human Research Protections (OHRP), the federal agency that oversees research on human subjects. In response to that complaint OHRP sent the Johns Hopkins Institutional Review Board (IRB) a frightening letter stating that they disagreed with Hopkins' interpretation that this work was exempt from IRB approval because it was quality improvement work, not human subjects research. The OHRP believed this was human subjects research. As such they claimed we had violated ethics rules because we did not obtain informed consent from patients. In addition, the agency said that we also needed approval from the IRBs at all the Michigan hospitals where our program had been implemented. The allegations were very serious, not just because they could put an end to our work but also because they could potentially prevent Johns Hopkins from receiving federal research dollars.

I was shocked and confused by the letter. I had submitted the proposal to the Johns Hopkins IRB and its members had concluded that it was not human subjects research but rather quality improvement. I had done exactly what I thought I was supposed to do. The IRB told us we did not need to obtain consent and approval from Michigan IRBs or Michigan patients. Well versed in research ethics, I fully agreed with the board's interpretation. While it was research, it was not human subjects research. The data that was collected did not contain any of the names of the participants; similarly, there was nothing in our program that could have put patients' confidentiality at risk. The Johns Hopkins IRB is exceedingly sophisticated and reviews over two thousand protocols a year. It seemed ridiculous that the OHRP, with little knowledge of what we actually did in the study, could make such conclusive statements. Our work posed little to no risk to patients. We were simply asking doctors to wash their hands, comply with national guidelines, improve teamwork, and monitor rates of infection—interventions that help rather than harm patients. If anything, these interventions substantially reduced risk; delaying its implementation posed far greater risks to patients.

But just as Waxman wielded serious power in Washington so did the OHRP. The letter caused an uproar; fear and trepidation rippled through the quality improvement community. Hospitals that had previously been interested in our work were now running for the hills, terrified. These institutions did not want the OHRP investigating, nor did they want the bad publicity that would accompany a sanction. Nobody wanted to see their hospital in the newspaper for violating ethics rules. What was most frightening for these hospitals was the capriciousness of the OHRP. If the OHRP had said, after the fact, that it did not like the way Hopkins' well-run and experienced IRB interpreted the rules, what would stop the OHRP from saying it did not like the interpretation of any hospital's IRB?

We were at a standstill. We had the money for the programs, but states would not participate until we clarified these issues with the OHRP. It looked like the project would never get off the ground. And worse yet, the OHRP demanded that we stop collecting data in Michigan.

My frustration led me to take a bold approach. I knew I needed to get in writing from the OHRP its exact position on the rules for this national effort before we started. I called the OHRP personally and spoke to the acting director, Ivor Pritchard. We had talked once at an Institute of Medicine Meeting and he seemed to understand our position and I believed he genuinely wanted to resolve the problem. I told him that we were poised to start implementing the project in more states and many of the hospitals did not have IRBs. I wanted him to put in writing whether or not this national effort qualified as human subjects research and required IRB approval. I didn't want to do all this work and then have the OHRP come at us again, late in the game, and tell us we had violated regulations. I wanted clearance ahead of time, in writing, so I could assure each hospital that it was safe to work with us.

As I expected, Ivor said that honoring my request would be difficult. He told me that the rules are complex and the OHRP generally does not issue written guidance. He said that he would be happy to talk to me, but he would not give me anything in writing. I felt trapped. I knew that hospitals would not sign up without this clarification from the OHRP and it was obvious that the OHRP was not going to offer that.

I might have been new to politics, but I was learning fast. I called my friend Stephen Cha in Waxman's office to explain the situation. Stephen was very angry at the OHRP's decision. He assured me that they would remedy the situation even if they had to schedule officials from the OHRP in for a hearing. Stephen assured me that he would also call Ivor personally to deliver the message. It was the first time I had been direct witness to Beltway power politics—it was both exciting and terrifying.

In the end, Ivor was very cooperative. We discussed the issues and developed a plan that was wise and just and he promised to send written guidelines for my review. I received the letter ten days later. It said that the participating hospitals were doing quality improvement work, not research, and that Hopkins was doing research, but it was not human subjects research.

I wanted to get a more general letter that would clarify the broader issue of disassociating quality improvement from human subjects research, as did many of my quality improvement colleagues. This would better guide and protect everyone who was doing or planned to do quality improvement work. I asked Ivor if that was possible, but he told me the OHRP could not issue such a sweeping letter in such short time. It would take substantial legal review. I did not want to compromise our program so Ivor and I agreed to focus only on our work to reduce central line infections.

Shortly after clearing this hurdle we got some good news from the Agency for Healthcare Research and Quality (AHRQ). A leader in the organization had found some money in the budget for our work. The only catch was the budget cycle was ending and the AHRQ had to use it before the cycle was over or lose it altogether. We would have loved it if they just gave us the cash, but that is not the way government works. In order to get that money, the AHRQ would have to allow a reasonable amount of time for organizations like ours to submit grants. The AHRQ would then need time to review them and decide—without any guarantees—that our project was best qualified for the money. This makes sense because it keeps government honest, or as honest as one can expect, but grants take time, so it looked like we were out of luck.

But then the people at the AHRQ came up with an idea. The Health Research and Education Trust (HRET)—a nonprofit subsidiary of the American Hospital Association that focuses on improving the delivery of health care—had already been approved to receive money. So it was decided that the AHRQ would give the money to the HRET and the HRET would work with our team and the Michigan Hospital Association to implement our program in ten states across the country. We chose to work with MHA because it had been such an integral part of our success in Michigan. The people there had also developed an excellent database I knew we would desperately need for this new project.

The HRET turned out to be a great strategic partner. The program required strong relationships with state hospital associations and since it was a part of the powerful American Hospital Association, the HRET had these relationships. As such, the group was indispensable for recruiting hospitals and state hospital associations. Moreover, the HRET staff loved and supported our model and believed in robust measurement.

With funding secured, we began strategizing. We decided to require that each state in our program have a strong centralized team with a director who could manage the state-based work. Our experience had taught us that the program was not sustainable without this kind of support and that the states each had to own the work of their hospitals.

We also had to beef up our Quality and Safety Research Group (QSRG) team. We needed more people and more time from the people we already had. The way it works in academic medicine is organizations like ours buy a percentage of a researcher's time. For most of our faculty, our grants and fellowships were paying for roughly 10 to 20 percent of their time. Increased funding allowed us to increase this effort substantially. We also added full-time project managers, data analysts, and research coordinators.

The money from the Sandlers and the anonymous donor combined with the AHRQ funding gave us enough money to work with twenty-eight states. From a management perspective, we broke into two groups along funding lines. The HRET and the MHA supported ten states, and my team, with philanthropy money, supported an additional eighteen. The QSRG was responsible for the content of the program—conducting the conference calls and the face-to-face meetings and supplying any and all the materials and information needed by the states. The HRET helped recruit hospitals and manage the program. And MHA managed the infection and culture data.

Things were looking good but, as always, we were concerned about getting valid, complete data. This had been a problem in almost every project we had run. So, as a preemptive strike, we sought out leverage from the private sector.

Consumers Union, the group that publishes *Consumer Reports*, also wanted to make these infection rates available to the public. However, as we know, many hospitals did not track these rates or, if they did, they were reluctant to publish them for fear of bad publicity. I figured that if I gave Consumers Union a list of the hospitals that were participating in our program, it would put pressure on other hospitals both to participate in the project and to measure rates. It was a tricky strategy because if I made publicly reporting infection rates mandatory, no states would sign up. Moreover, it is the states' data, not ours, and we do not have the authority to make their data public. However, simply by sharing the list of participating hospitals with Consumers Union and letting it exercise its subtle and not so subtle pressure, we would be well enough distanced and it wouldn't interfere with our work.

To the same purpose, we also formed a partnership with the Leapfrog Group, the organization that first invited me to Michigan to discuss my research on placing intensivist in the ICU. This consortium of more than one hundred Fortune 500 companies that buy health care for tens of millions of employees has significant leverage with insurers and hospitals. The Leapfrog Group conducts regular national surveys of hospitals to find out which ones are meeting its standards. After reading the Government Accountability Office report and hearing about our success in wiping out these infections, Leapfrog's CEO, Leah Binder, decided to ask the hospitals in the survey to report their ICU central line infection rates. She also decided to give credit to hospitals participating in our project.

In addition, the Joint Commission made reducing bloodstream infections one of its national patient safety goals, in part based on our Michigan work. The interventions the Joint Commission asked hospitals to do are robust, practical, and evidence-based; they address leadership responsibilities, infection control, and ICU practices. They include all the elements needed to effectively reduce these infections. Making these interventions part of the Joint Commission's national patient safety goals means that hospitals that don't comply are ineligible for Medicare funding to pay for the cost of related care due to bloodstream infections. This could easily put a hospital out of business. Although the Joint Commission is a private sector, nonprofit organization, it has been granted the power to make these calls. Hospitals must be accredited by the Joint Commission to receive Medicare dollars.

We also partnered with the Centers for Disease Control and Prevention, which has traditionally been in charge of measuring and reducing these infections on a national level. The CDC people agreed to make their technical experts available to our teams and states. They also agreed to collaborate on collecting data so that we could make it easier and more practical for resource-constrained hospitals. In addition they agreed to connect us to state health departments, which are often charged with collecting infection data for states. Finally, they connected us with state-based quality improvement organizations, which monitor the quality of care for the Center for Medicare and Medicaid Services (CMS). This marked the first time public health efforts were linked with quality improvement.

With philanthropic money, AHRQ funding, senators and congresspeople lending a hand and these powerful private sector organizations backing us up, we were ready to get to work. Little did we know our world was about to double in size.

Our efforts in Michigan and Washington had gotten the attention of the new secretary of Health and Human Services, Kathleen Sebelius. Referring to our work, she called for a 75 percent reduction in ICU bloodstream infections within three years in all U.S. hospitals. This was the first time there was an empiric, measurable national goal for improving health care quality. In addition, Obama's newly formed Office of Health Reform issued a report on our Michigan work, calling it a success story.

On the heels of that announcement the AHRQ contacted the HRET and said it had more money and wanted us to expand our project to more states. This added funding enabled us to do the entire country, coast to coast, Alaska and Hawaii, and even Puerto Rico. Twenty-eight states is good, but clearly it is not enough. As long as there is one hospital where people are dying needlessly because of a preventable central line infection, it is unacceptable. We needed to be able to say that every American is safe from central line infections at every hospital in the entire United States, be it a small regional hospital or a large academic center. And eliminating these infections is only the beginning. There are a multitude of similar defects in medicine that cause harm to patients. And we are confident that our system of checklists, culture change, and measurement will be equally effective at tackling these problems as well.

The dominoes that we had been waiting for were starting to fall and I could barely keep up with them. According to one of Johns Hopkins' health care lobbyists, we had started a buzz on Capitol Hill. We tried to keep our message simple, science based, and focused on the patient, not on policy. Washington liked this message. Moreover everyone agreed that reducing infections must be partnered with improving culture, and that our efforts required valid data behind it so that it could be accountable to the public.

Only a few years back we were a small team struggling to reduce bloodstream infections in the Hopkins ICU. Now there was a growing army of like-minded patients and safety soldiers all working together toward a common goal. As this team expanded, so did the scope of our work. As exciting as it was to see our program reduce bloodstream infections spreading across the country, we had other projects that also desperately needed federal funding. So we turned once again to our new colleagues in Washington hoping to expand this support and the patient safety movement.

# Chapter 9

In addition to my testimony in front of Waxman's hearing, I was asked to testify in front of the Senate Committee on Health, Education, Labor and Pensions chaired by Senator Edward Kennedy. The HELP Committee had a working group on quality of care chaired by Senator Mikulski. I saw this as a perfect opportunity to address some of our other patient safety initiatives.

One of these initiatives addresses the need for a federal program that helps medicine learn from its mistakes. Currently there is no national infrastructure enabling health care as a whole to learn from common, costly, and lethal mistakes that are beyond the capacity of any single health system to fix. Consider an error that recently occurred to a patient who was undergoing knee replacement surgery. The doctors elected to use an epidural catheter, rather than intravenous narcotics, to provide pain relief. Epidural catheters are commonly used to ease the pain during labor and are also used in certain surgical procedures. Unlike the central line catheter, which goes directly into a patient's bloodstream, medicines transmitted through epidural catheters are released into the epidural space—a space that is separated from the spinal fluid by a cellophanelike membrane. The medicine slowly leeches through this membrane into the spinal

fluid. Due to a poor design, the connector on the epidural catheter is
identical to the connector on an intravenous catheter. They even use
the same tubing. Predictably, the nurse hooked the medication up
to the patient's intravenous catheter and delivered the drug directly
into her bloodstream. Luckily the patient suffered no harm, but she
could have. Some pain medications we inject into the epidural space
can kill if administered directly into the bloodstream. Data from
hospital error-reporting systems suggests this mistake occurs multiple times per year in all six thousand U.S. hospitals. And these
estimates are probably on the low side—on average, error-reporting
systems identify only one of every twenty events.

Hopkins created a team to investigate and mitigate the risk of
this error. The team recognized that the optimal solution was to design the two catheters with different connectors so this could not
happen again. However, a single hospital or even a large system does
not have the financial or political leverage to get manufacturers to
redesign their catheters. So the team members did what they could
do. They created a hospitalwide campaign to aggressively educate
staff about the dangers of this error.

These types of educational campaigns occur commonly throughout hospitals. Yet we know from experience and from safety experts
in a variety of industries that education alone does little to improve
safety. Humans are fallible and rather ingenious at finding ways to
put things together that do not belong together. If it remains possible to connect the catheters incorrectly, doctors and nurses will
continue to do it the wrong way.

It is also not a cost-effective approach. We know this mistake
occurs in all U.S. hospitals. Assume that every hospital embarks on
a similar program to reeducate staff—the class takes about an hour
and must be repeated annually. There are approximately 2 million

nurses working in the United States. To make the math easy, let's assume the average nurse earns approximately $50 per hour with benefits. That means the U.S. health system would have to spend $100 million a year, not including the cost to reeducate physicians, on a program that has close to a zero probability of working.

This example is but one of scores of risks to patients in which the "therapy" is simply to reeducate clinicians. There are things individual hospitals can do to make patients safe, but simply telling staff to "be more careful" is not one of them.

Obviously the solution that makes the most sense and is likely the most cost-effective is to redesign the catheters so that they cannot connect. This is exactly what anesthesiologists did decades ago to prevent accidentally hooking an oxygen hose up to a nitrous oxide feed. That mistake, which used to kill patients, has been eliminated because the hoses were redesigned—at a cost of far less than $100 million. Unfortunately, success stories like this are rare. We need to change that. We need a system that identifies sensible, practical solutions like these and propagates them throughout the health system. To accomplish this we will need to gain enough leverage to influence device manufacturers to make changes. Hospitals can't do this alone; they need a structure to convene public and private organizations as well as the power and financial support of government.

Long ago the aviation industry struggled with this same problem. They concluded it was foolish to have individual airlines investigate and learn from mistakes in isolation. They formed a public private partnership called the Commercial Aviation Safety Team (CAST). CAST brings together the entire airline industry—major airline manufacturers, airline companies, labor organizations, government agencies such as the Federal Aviation Administration, and international organizations such as the Flight Safety Foundation.

These groups work together to prioritize the industry's greatest risks, investigate them thoroughly, and design and implement interventions that work. Since its founding in 1997, CAST has helped the aviation industry improve an already admirable record of safety. Between 1994 and 2004, the average rate of fatal accidents decreased from 0.05 to 0.02 per 100,000 departures, largely due to these efforts. In CUSP we reduce the risk from defects on a unit level but not on a national level. We need a CAST for health care that will investigate defects thoroughly and design and implement interventions that work not just in one hospital, but in all hospitals across the country.

A second national patient safety initiative that we knew must have federal guidance and support is the need for valid measurement and accurate reporting of health care quality and safety. Imagine that the United States was confronted with a deadly disease, and that this disease had claimed approximately 1 million lives over the last quarter century—twice as many as have died from AIDS. A group of researchers developed a treatment that would effectively wipe out the disease across the nation, saving more lives than virtually any other medical discovery in the past twenty-five years.

That disease is central line infection and the treatment is our checklist. Yet, this treatment is not being used, and people continue to die. Why? Because like many errors in health care, they happen inside the hospital and rates are not reported, so they are invisible to the public.

A patient is admitted, the curtain is drawn, and what goes on behind that curtain is murky and often secretive. If someone does not wash his hands and infects the patient, it's likely nobody else sees it or nobody reports it. When that patient suffers a complication, it's chalked up as the cost of caring for the sick and dying.

When a patient dies from a central line infection a doctor doesn't step forward and tell the family, "I'm sorry, I didn't wear a mask and gown when placing his central line catheter; I gave your loved one an infection that killed him. If I had taken the proper precautions, he would still be alive." Doctors don't say this because doctors don't make mistakes. They do the best they can and if a patient dies they believe it's because some people make it and some don't. Deaths and complications are often deemed acts of God. All physicians are ac-culturated to accept this fact. Perhaps it is a defense mechanism; if physicians were not able to compartmentalize their mistakes they would not likely be able to handle the emotional strain of treating patients day in and day out.

But we have shown that central line infections are not inevitable; they are preventable. They are usually the result of system errors and poor culture. Still, this message has not reached the public or arrived at the bedside; we are still operating in the dark and the patient suf-fers. Waxman's survey revealed that while all states said they were using the checklist, only eleven states monitored infection rates, and few, if any, had rates as low as Michigan's. If we could guarantee accurate reporting of these infection rates and make these numbers available to consumers and legislators, we would raise awareness and hospitals would be more likely to implement interventions to reduce these infections. I have no doubt that if all hospitals were required to have a sign in front of the entrance that accurately reported their central line infection rates, hospitals would rapidly adopt the pro-gram and dramatically reduce these infections.

We need a government-based agency that not only demands that hospitals measure and track safety records—such as bloodstream infection rates—but that also regulates these measures to ensure they are uniform and accurate. In 1934, the United States created the Securities and Exchange Commission (SEC) to bring this level of transparency and accuracy to financial reporting. Prior to 1934, consumers were at great risk from misinformation and marginal financiers who promised impossible returns on investment. The most infamous of these was a man named Charles Ponzi, who bilked the public out of millions of dollars using a system that—if regulated—would have been quickly exposed as a fraud.

Ponzi promised a 100 percent return on investment in only ninety days. He achieved these returns by attracting enough new investors to pay off the few that cashed in early. His scheme was supported by the fact that most of his investors left their "profits" "invested" so that the money would continue to "grow." Yet not a single dime invested with Ponzi ever generated any profit. At that time there was no governmental body, or any other organization, that investigated financial entrepreneurs or guaranteed financial statements were accurate.

The exposure of Ponzi's deceit, the eventual collapse of numerous prominent banks, and other factors led to a decision by Franklin Delano Roosevelt to create the SEC. The SEC ensured the accuracy of financial data and substantially enhanced the efficiency of markets. It created rules known as generally accepted accounting principles that mandated and governed financial reporting. It created a whole new profession of certified public accountants who knew the rules, were trained in measurement, provided accountability by auditing performance, and imposed stiff fines for violations.

Of course, the SEC is not perfect; crafty financiers such as Michael Milken and Bernie Madoff, as well as corporations such as Enron and WorldCom, have successfully deceived the public despite the best efforts of the SEC. However, the commission has undoubtedly protected the public from hundreds if not thousands of other potential financial scams over the years. Furthermore, it has been very effective at ensuring transparency in financial reporting. As a result, the financial markets are much more efficient because of these regulations.

The parallels between health care and finance are striking. Both depend on having up-to-date and complete information. When the information isn't correct or current, people make bad decisions and the consumer suffers. The mortgage crisis happened because homeowners were permitted to take out mortgages that would eventually exceed their monthly income. This was further compounded by well-intended federal policies that encouraged home ownership. Investors bought these mortgages not knowing they were worthless. If consumers and investors had been provided with accurate information on what they were buying and the potential risks, everyone would have made better decisions and the collapse would have been avoided. It's clear that many bad decisions in both health care and finance result from the lack of accurate, timely information.

Sometimes the problem is not so much a lack of information as an overload of complex and often exaggerated or misleading information. As a result, most ordinary people—even some experts—are unable to sift through this pile of confusing statistics and identify the credible information they need to guide choices and make good decisions.

In health care we are inundated with claims about "quality of care" but given little accurate data. We have few standards for gathering such information and even fewer guidelines that help ordinary people understand what the information means. Health care desperately needs trained professionals to create standardized regulations for reporting, audits to ensure the reports are accurate, and penalties for those who digress.

As a result of this absence of oversight on safety reporting, hospitals advertise erroneous and misleading information on Web sites, in glossy brochures, on billboards, and on TV. There is no assurance of the accuracy of their claims, because the measurement of quality in health care is neither standardized nor consistently reliable. Indeed, hospital reports about quality of care are held to no higher standard than the advertising of toothpaste or washing machines.

One hospital Web site reported that patients should come to that institution because it had saved 242 lives during an eighteen-month period. But it was unclear how the hospital had made this estimate—what kind of patients were counted or how many were studied. Another hospital Web site claimed that it had screened and given pneumococcal vaccinations to 94 percent of eligible patients, whereas a government Web site (www.hospitalcompare.hhs.gov) on the same day reported that only 64 percent of patients at that hospital were vaccinated. Another hospital vaguely reported that it had zero infections, implying that patients would not be infected if they sought care there. Yet it did not offer any indication of how it had arrived at this conclusion, what types of infections were included, or for how long the rate was measured—one week, one month, a year, or five years?

Similarly, profit-oriented private enterprises that report on the quality of care are completely unregulated. Since their rating methods are proprietary, opaque, and generally more promotional than scientific, they frequently misinform or confuse the public. For example, not one hospital made it on all three of the major hospital ranking lists: the *U.S. News and World Report*, HealthGrades, and J. D. Power and Associates. If these agencies are accurately measuring hospital quality, how can that be? Some companies often create lists of "best hospitals" and "best doctors" and then turn around and sell services to the very hospitals listed as top performers. Others only include a hospital in their lists if the institution purchases their services. This is eerily similar to the concerns raised about bond rating agencies being paid by the companies whose products they evaluate, yet much more flagrant.

Such incomplete or misleading reports about quality-of-care measures pose significant risks to patients, clinicians, and insurance companies. Patients might choose care according to misinformation and make poor decisions. Health care organizations may become overconfident about the quality of care provided, reduce or eliminate improvement efforts, and increase the risks of preventable harm. Insurers may mistakenly channel patients to overrated, low-quality clinicians or overestimate or underestimate the benefits of certain procedures.

The public deserves better. Public reporting of quality measures should have at least the same reporting standards as the reporting of financial data: explicit rules regarding what data to collect, trained professionals to oversee data collection, and regular auditing and enforcement of data integrity standards. Hospitals or other organizations that gather, report, and publicize health care quality measures must be held accountable for their accuracy.

At the very least, the federal government should do for health care what it began to do in 1934 for financial data—ensure its accuracy and transparency so that health care services can truly compete on quality. The U.S. public deserves to know that the information they have about hospital quality and safety is accurate and timely.

The third initiative we introduced in my testimony has been key to our mission since day one—the creation of a government body whose sole purpose is to support research in patient safety and quality of care. At present, our government invests little in helping improve the systems we use to deliver new treatments to the bedside. Getting quality and safety research accepted as legitimate in academic medical centers so we can address this problem is a challenge. There are few physicians with training to conduct robust safety research and few promotions committees in academic medical centers that recognize this work. Winning the MacArthur helped, but it will likely take a safety researcher winning the Nobel Prize to legitimize our work. Unfortunately, even that is unlikely since the Nobel in Medicine is still mostly geared toward discoveries in the lab rather than to innovations in patient care or safety. Our goal is to change this paradigm so patient safety and patient care research is conducted and viewed on an equal scientific playing field as work performed in a lab or test tube. Our central line infection studies were one of the first patient safety studies conducted under the same scientific rigor as a drug test or any other clinical trial.

In phase 1, we reviewed existing data and selected five key procedures that would most likely prevent these infections. We compiled these procedures into an easy-to-follow checklist. We identified potential barriers to using the checklist and developed tactics to overcome those barriers so we could optimize compliance. We then pilot-tested the intervention at Johns Hopkins and measured performance. The result was that we nearly eliminated these infections.

In phase 2, AHRQ provided a matching grant to help us pilot test the program in the state of Michigan. Within three months of implementing the interventions, we nearly eliminated these infections in all of the 103 participating ICUs; it has stayed that way for four years. The work was not easy; it required hospital leaders, doctors, and nurses to implement interventions, improve teamwork, and monitor performance. But the results were well worth the investment. In just one year, the reduction in infections was estimated to have saved the hospital system millions of dollars, two hundred dollars for every dollar invested, and thousands of lives.

In phase 3, we are trying to implement this program across the United States, state by state, hospital by hospital. Thanks to funding from AHRQ, we are implementing this life-saving program across the country. Most states are trying to reduce these infections, but they need support in order to be efficient, and to rigorously measure and improve performance.

Having our results recognized and published by the *New England Journal of Medicine* has helped the world to understand that patient safety research is as much a science as biomedical research. And just as biomedical research depends on the NIH, we need a similar federal institution to help support continued patient safety research. That's not to say we should borrow from or cut the NIH budget; it's essential that we keep learning how to better treat diseases. But if we are not investing equally in methods for getting these new treatments to the bedside, we are only halfway toward making patients healthier. An institute would not only help direct funding, but it could also help organize global efforts to improve safety. There is a tremendous amount of work to do. Bloodstream infections is just one of hundreds, if not thousands, of hospital errors that harm patients or squander resources. This institute would help us achieve the common goal of addressing these serious patient safety concerns and in turn greatly improve the health of America's citizens.

With all of this running through my mind I climbed the marble steps of the Dirksen Senate Office Building. All the conversations we had been having with politicians had really honed my message. And they had given me insights into what moves the political machine. I knew I had to tell rich stories peppered with facts if I wanted to keep the attention of this audience. And I was fairly confident that what I was going to say would hit some chords with the committee.

As I presented our case in front of this handful of powerful senators it was hard to tell if I was getting through. Their behavior at these hearings makes them resemble a person with chronic attention deficit disorder. They are constantly getting calls or text messages, their staff pass them notes or whisper in their ears, and they continuously get up and leave in the middle of a presentation, sometimes never returning. I felt fairly inadequate sitting there, talking to this restless, overly stimulated, distracted audience. However, when I finished I saw the chamber spring to life. Senators' heads were nodding as if they had connected with what I had said and were eager to comment.

Senator Kay Hagan from North Carolina was the first to speak up. She thanked me for my comments. And then she became quizzical and incredulous, saying that she wanted to know how it was possible we had figured out how to make diesel fuel nozzles that don't fit gas-powered cars, but we can't figure out how to make different types of catheter connections so doctors don't place patients in harm's way. It was a perfect analogy, in fact one that I use today. I was relieved; my message was getting through.

Senator Sherrod Brown sat up and perched himself on the edge of his chair. Almost as an extension of our previous meeting, he reiterated the importance of ending bloodstream infections across the United States. He added that our system provided a clear path toward reaching that goal. He also thanked Senator Hagan for her contributions and agreed with her on the need for a CAST for health care.

Senator Mikulski, who was chairing the committee, also chimed in with support for both a health care CAST and my checklist. She asked me how I thought my work would help her neighbor who has diabetes and who perhaps drinks too many beers and eats too many crabs. I laughed and told her that just as we had created a check-list for central line infections, we could easily create a checklist for diabetes or for any disease or procedure. The same principles would apply and likely we would get the same results. All we needed was support from the federal government and there was no limit to what we could achieve.

In closing she said, "Thank you so much; this seems so simple, we have to do this. It saves lives and dollars."

After the hearing Senator Mikulski came up to me, shook my hand, and told me she had read a lot about my work and was very proud of what our team had accomplished, especially since we came from her home state. She said she was going to work hard to build support for our ideas and was going to visit Hopkins soon to talk about her plan.

In spite of the excitement I had at this hearing, I tried to be re-alistic. I didn't expect anything to move very quickly on any of these fronts and I tried to absorb these proceedings with a grain or two of salt—these were politicians, after all, and politicians have a lot on their plates. Was I ever wrong.

A couple of weeks later I got an excited call from Senator Mikul-ski's main health care staffer. Mikulski was going to place a provi-sion within the Senate's national health care reform bill to establish an Office of Patient Safety Research to "identify and disseminate the best ideas and the best practices that save lives and save money— and make sure they are used in clinical training and practice."

She sent me a draft of the bill, which I reviewed with Marlene and Chris, and I sent back comments. A month later, she came to Johns Hopkins Hospital and held a press conference to announce the bill. Ed Miller introduced Senator Mikulski, who in turn introduced me—a kind gesture that took me by surprise. She had clearly taken me under her wing as a trusted adviser on patient safety and I was both humbled and honored. When these discussions had wrapped up, she announced her health care bill. It reads:

WASHINGTON, D.C.—U.S. Senator Barbara A. Mikulski (D-Md.) today announced she has included a provision within the Senate's national health care reform bill to make innovations like the Pronovost Checklist developed at Johns Hopkins Medicine available to improve lives, save lives and save money nationally.

"Health care must not only be available but affordable," said Senator Mikulski, a senior member of the Health, Education, Labor and Pensions (HELP) Committee and Chairwoman of the HELP workgroup on quality. "One way to make health care affordable is to deliver better quality and safety. Safety measures save lives and save money."

As author of the quality title of HELP's health care reform bill, the Affordable Health Choices Act, Senator Mikulski established an Office of Patient Safety Research to identify and disseminate the best ideas and the best practices that save lives and save money—and make sure they are used in clinical training and practice. Improvements in patient safety present an enormous opportunity for improving health care and reducing costs. Medical errors likely kill hundreds of thousands of people and cost America's health system billions of dollars each year.

The Pronovost Checklist, developed by Peter J. Pronovost, M.D., Ph.D., Sc.D., Johns Hopkins Medicine, is an exemplary example of a low-cost, low-tech solution that has a high impact on improving patient safety. It is a 5-step checklist that guides health care teams in properly inserting central lines that has been shown to reduce bloodstream infections related to these catheters.

When used for 18 months in Michigan hospitals, the Checklist saved 1,500 lives and saved $175 million. If used in hospitals nationwide, the Pronovost Checklist could save between $5 billion and $10 billion a year in the cost of treating avoidable complications.

"We've heard about Dr. Pronovost's checklists from learned journals and from the TV show *ER*," Senator Mikulski said. "They have spoken about a low-cost, low-tech solution that has a high impact. Dr. Peter Pronovost was first to recognize checklists have power to save lives and save money."

The Office for Patient Safety Research will be housed within the Agency for Healthcare Research and Quality at the Department of Health and Human Services. Its experts will research how to deliver best practices safely and efficiently, develop mechanisms for setting national priorities in quality, research how to improve delivery of health care, design interventions to prevent medical mistakes, and develop programs to translate evidence into practice. It also will provide grants to identify and disseminate best practices, like the Pronovost Checklist, to providers and patients across the country.

After Senator Mikulski had made her announcement she asked me to come up and say a few words. I thanked her, expressed my gratitude for her support for patient safety research, and reiterated the desperate need for this level of support. This was an important moment for our work and for Hopkins. This high-profile event only further illustrated to me, my colleagues, Hopkins leadership, and the nation that patient safety awareness was clearly on the rise; a new science was emerging, a science that now had credibility and financial support.

It was an exciting time for our team. Conversations that began among colleagues at Hopkins had captured the attention of congresspeople, senators, and other world leaders. We had helped motivate an international patient safety learning community that contained some of the brightest doctors, nurses, human factors engineers, social scientists, epidemiologists, anthropologists, biostatisticians, and informatics experts in medicine. Safety research is now a legitimate scientific discipline and there is more demand for patient safety from the health care community than we could have ever imagined. But what does this mean to the average patient walking through the doors of Johns Hopkins Hospital, where this work first began? Is this patient actually safer?

# Chapter 10

===

Let's examine four relatively common diseases that likely touch everyone's life either personally or through a loved one—cancer, mental illness, heart disease, and stroke. With each of these diseases I will try to demonstrate patient safety efforts have either directly or indirectly made the patient experience better from admission to discharge to outpatient care.

Our first example is an imaginary patient we will call James. James is in his fifties and has gone to his primary care physician because he has been feeling tired and depressed, has some abdominal pain, and has recently lost a lot of weight. He is recommended to a specialist at Johns Hopkins. Our work begins with the diagnosis. If James has pancreatic cancer but it is misdiagnosed, as it commonly is, it could spread to other parts of the body such as the liver, the lungs, and the bile duct (a tube that delivers bile from the liver to the small intestines). Once the cancer has metastasized, it is almost impossible to save the patient. Therefore, as is true with most cancers, early diagnosis of pancreatic cancer is the key to survival. (Early and correct diagnosis of my father's cancer would have most likely saved his life, so this issue is especially close to my heart.)

Our best estimates suggest that misdiagnosis kills at least forty thousand to eighty thousand people every year (although this is likely a gross underestimation). Patients are harmed from the delay or failure to treat a condition that was missed, or when a physician treats a condition the patient doesn't actually have. Misdiagnosis is one of the relatively unexplored areas of potential patient harm and one of the most devastating in terms of cost, death, and injury. Diagnostic errors are more than three times more likely to result in serious disability than drug errors. However, the majority of diagnostic errors are both unrecognized and unreported. The science of how to measure and reduce these errors is grossly underdeveloped.

We are applying our theories of improved communication and culture to help reduce misdiagnosis. The *Journal of the American Medical Association* recently published a paper I coauthored in which we demonstrated that physicians often rely too heavily on their own limited knowledge regarding a particular illness. In this way they are often blind to, or unaware of, the wealth of knowledge contained in the medical literature or the expertise of colleagues in the field. This is due in part to ego and autonomy, but also to the lack of any effective system for sharing and distributing this knowledge. We are looking at ways to change that model, to deliver the latest diagnostic and therapeutic techniques into the hands of all doctors throughout the world.

Luckily James consults Johns Hopkins cancer surgeon Dr. Rich Schulick—a CUSP champion whom I work with on Weinberg-4C. Rich, realizing the value of diverse and independent input, consults his team, gathers all available information and resources at his disposal, and makes the correct diagnosis. He schedules James for surgery—the most common and most effective treatment for this type of disease.

James arrives on the morning of his surgery and goes first to the post-anesthesia care unit (PACU). There, thanks to the CUSP initiative of medication reconciliation, the physicians and nurses will be clear on what medications James has taken in the past, is currently taking, and will receive during surgery. The doctors and nurses will also discuss James's medical history with his family. In the past there was no clear system for medication reconciliation, meaning valuable information from the family that might not be in the chart could be lost or inaccurate. It also meant that James's medical history might not have been shared with the other members of the care team. When we first started our safety efforts we found that in 75 percent of cases, the surgeons, anesthesiologists, and patients did not agree on what medication the patient was taking. These lapses could easily result in treatment errors and potential harm to our patient. Thanks to efforts to improve safety, this problem has been virtually eliminated.

Next in the PACU, the surgeon physically marks the area on the body where he is going to make his first incision—one of the interventions designed to prevent wrong-site surgery. Once James has been wheeled into the operating room, a central line may be placed. Since we extended the ICU program used to reduce central line infections to the operating room and emergency department—where many central lines are placed—the anesthesiologist would wash her hands; use a gown, mask, gloves, and chlorhexidine antiseptic; and avoid the femoral site. She would also discuss with the surgeon whether the central line was even needed.

Before surgery begins, the physicians will also decide whether or not James needs a urinary catheter—a tube placed in his urethra that leads to a bag that collects urine. This came out of a CUSP initiative that recognized that these catheters should only be used when absolutely necessary because they present a potential risk. Urinary catheters help a physician assess the volume of fluid in the patient by measuring how much fluid comes out and comparing it with how much goes in via an IV or a central line catheter (for example). This volume is directly tied to the health of various organs like the kidneys and the heart and is an especially important indicator for patients who have already bled a lot due to injury or who will lose blood during the operation—for example, cardiac surgery patients.

The risk is that urinary catheters—like all catheters—can cause serious infection. These infections are either introduced when the catheter is placed without proper sterile procedures, or they occur if it is left in too long. Urinary tract infections, especially in young patients, can cause kidney scarring, which can result in kidney failure later in life. Though they are unlikely to kill, they are the most common type of hospital-acquired infection and they cause discomfort, prolonged hospital stay, and excess costs of care.

In spite of this risk, however, there was no protocol for placing these catheters nor was there a clear directive for removing them when they were not longer necessary. Today that has all changed. Catheters are only used when deemed necessary for a specific procedure. We also put in place a checklist—similar to what we use when placing central lines—to combat infection. Finally, we have a second checklist that requires these catheters be removed as soon as they are no longer necessary—usually the first day after surgery, when the patient is stable and ready to leave the ICU. Because James's surgery is a large operation that will take some time, the surgery residents place a catheter, using all the necessary precautions.

Before James's surgeon makes the first incision, the team conducts a surgery briefing. Aside from adding clarity to the procedure, briefings like this have really helped create a positive culture in the operating room. The briefing is a simple but effective expansion of the Joint Commission's required time-out safety initiative (which was more focused on technical problems than cultural issues). In the past, likely because culture was not addressed, surgeons would simply ignore the time-out. A nurse would often sit in a corner reviewing the case out loud, but nobody would be listening or necessarily even be in the room.

Today the briefing is led by Rich and everyone who will be in the operating room must be present. James's briefing takes place at seven a.m. in the operating room. The entire surgery team is there, James has been put under, and Rich is ready to start cutting. Before knife hits skin Rich introduces himself, by his first name and his role, and asks the other team members to do the same. Everyone's name and role is written on a whiteboard on the wall of the operating room. In some operating rooms, there is an LCD screen that displays the information.

Rich has published several papers on improving culture in the operating room and is a true leader in the field. Having respected surgeons like Rich participate and support these safety initiatives is key to the advancement of our work. As Rich teaches young residents and medical students how to perform complex surgical procedures, he is also teaching them teamwork and good culture. Without support from physicians like Rich, our work would collapse.

The patient, James, is identified correctly and the surgery marking is confirmed. The name of the procedure is posted and double-checked for accuracy. The surgeon confirms the antibiotics have been administered, noting the patient's penicillin allergy. The surgeon continues by describing the surgical steps of the procedure and notes when the potential problems could occur; he asks the team members if they have any concerns about the patient's safety they want to discuss. He asks the team members, if something were to go wrong in this case, what would it be and how could he defend against it. He also adds, "If anyone sees anything during this case that doesn't look right, please let me know."

Next, the anesthesiologist discusses James's starting hemoglobin level and also confirms that James's blood is in good supply in the blood bank should he need it. She then explains what she will be doing during the surgery and any concerns she has, so everyone is on the same page. Furthermore she tells the team that James has no significant medical problems that pose risks for him and that he will be going to the WICU after surgery and that the bed has been confirmed.

A nurse performs an inventory of all the surgical instruments and equipment required for the procedure. She explains that one of her peers will be taking her place in two hours. The surgeon reiterates that team members should speak up if they see any problems and confirms that everyone is ready to proceed. After this process is completed, and only then, does the surgeon make the incision.

In the past, much of this would not have happened. The surgeon would have likely come into the operating room, maybe said a few words, though most often said nothing, and started cutting. He might not have known half the names of the people in the room. Anesthesiologists and nurses might hint or make suggestions if they were concerned, but they would likely not directly and openly address risks. No wonder wrong-site surgery and other errors were so common.

Introducing members of the operating room team and encouraging them to speak openly and freely creates a much healthier work climate. It has been shown in business meetings that once a person has been given the opportunity to speak, that person is more likely to speak up again during the meeting. Similarly, by introducing everyone and opening the floor up for discussion, nurses and the anesthesiologist are more likely to alert the surgeon if they sense something is not quite right.

These local culture improvements, collectively, have a powerful effect on the institution. When nurses or doctors witness better communication and teamwork between them, it creates a buzz that quickly spreads through the hallways, break rooms, and cafeterias in the hospital. When you have top executives backing these types of changes, it adds even more power to these discussions. Similarly, we now give the science of safety talk to all new residents, making sure they understand that this science-based work does as much to save lives as anything they will learn in the classroom or on the unit. When these young residents travel through many different parts of the hospital and get exposed to our work by safety champions like Rich, it only further cements their patient safety training. When the residents eventually graduate into faculty positions, gain power, and take leadership positions, they will look at the roles of nurses, physicians, and patients in a different light, thanks to what they have seen, heard, and learned. These doctors will understand that they don't lose power by listening to coworkers no matter where anyone's place is in the hierarchy. It takes time and patience to change the way we do things, to change culture. But we are doing it, one unit, one surgeon, and one nurse at a time.

When James's surgery is completed, the entire team holds a debriefing. Nurses count and verify the numbers of sponges, needles, and instruments to make sure nothing was left inside James (which was previously a very common error). The surgeon also confirms the correct labeling of any specimens collected during surgery—another very common error that can have devastating consequences. If tissue samples get mixed up in the lab, who knows what treatments could be erroneously recommended for the patient?

Finally, the surgeon talks to the team about what they thought went well and what could have been done better. He then appoints a member of the team to be the leader in making changes to fix whatever problems were identified.

Programs that identify errors before they happen are new to hospitals and long overdue. Frankly it's hard to fathom why we didn't have systems like this in place before. It seems an obvious safety precaution. When my son, Ethan, was a toddler and first became mobile, my wife, Marlene, and I went around the house and identified areas of potential harm. We proactively removed breakable items, put gates at the top of stairs, and put cushions over sharp edges. It was common sense. Yet for some reason, hospitals (which have far more potential dangers than our house) have never viewed this as important. They react well when something goes wrong, but by then it is often too late; patients have already been harmed or killed. It's surprising that they haven't developed eyes to see things before that harm occurs.

This debriefing might sound cumbersome. And to be honest, some surgeons probably see it as a waste of time. But there was also a time when surgeons thought it was a waste of time to put on surgical gloves, gowns, or masks in the operating room. But like gowns, gloves, and masks, the debriefing, and all the safety work we do, is supported by evidence. It has been tested and measured and proven to make patients safer.

After the debriefing, James is wheeled into the WICU. One of our most important safety initiatives applies whenever a patient changes units—the handoff. There is a lot of very important information that the new team needs from the prior team. Yet in the past, with no clear system for handoffs, much of this information was lost. Sloppy handoffs pose huge risks for patients. Forgotten or inaccurate information can cause harm or even kill.

Today, we have a handoff sheet that is reviewed by both the sending and the receiving teams. It includes all the important medical information regarding the care plan as well as specific details about the patient's particular needs. As James enters the WICU, clinicians will discuss any significant events that happened in the operating room. They will review his medical history and ensure he is getting medicine to prevent blood clots, a complication that kills more than 400,000 people a year, and medicine to prevent stomach ulcers—all of this driven by our CUSP work and checklists.

The care team uses our urinary catheter checklist and determines James no longer needs his, so it is removed after one night in the WICU to prevent possible infection. Similarly, if James needs to be ventilated he will receive all the precautions contained in the VAP checklist. Nurses and physicians will wash hands before and after entering his room to ensure that James doesn't acquire a deadly infection from another patient. In addition, if a patient comes onto the unit infected with a bacterial infection, the ICU staff will be notified of this infection prior to the infected patient's arrival and plan accordingly. Every staff member will wear proper barrier protection before going into contaminated rooms to further protect James and the other patients on the unit. None of this happened in the past.

To make sure everyone on the floor knows exactly what the care plan is for James, they all make rounds together and use the daily goals sheet to clarify that plan. Furthermore, James's family can be present during the rounds and is encouraged to review and discuss the plan for his care. There are twenty-four/seven visiting hours for his family members so they can be close to James and be part of the care team. If James needs to stay in the ICU for a long time, we would schedule more formal weekly family meetings to discuss James's current status, prognosis, and goals of care.

Having families present when the team makes its rounds, what we call family-centered care, is one of our new initiatives that we are very proud of. The director of surgical nursing, Deb Baker, is a champion of this new care program and she is working to put it in every surgical unit in the hospital. She recently told me of the family of a sixteen-year-old child who had severe brain injury from an automobile accident and was going to die. The patient had been hospitalized prior to the expanded visiting hours. Back then, the parents were limited to only a couple of hours to visit with their son. Furthermore, the waiting area had a sign on it that said WAITING AREA CLOSES AT 12 A.M. And although it is likely nurses would bend the rules and let family members see their dying son, it still creates an environment that does not support patient-centered care.

It is not enough just to care for the patient; you also need to care for the family. Plus, as Sorrel King taught us, a physician can learn a lot about a patient by listening to the family. Physicians and nurses need to stop seeing families as interference, but as an opportunity to improve patient care. It has been shown that patient outcomes improve when patients and their families more actively participate. It is also a moral imperative to involve patients and their families in the care. It's the right thing to do. Yet in much of medicine, they are not made to feel welcome on the unit. As caregivers, we often seem to forget that we are visitors in their world.

After the patient is released from the WICU he moves down to Weinberg-4C. Once again, handoff forms and medication reconciliation procedures will apply. Once James arrives at Weinberg-4C, he will benefit from another CUSP initiative, patient cohorting—patients with similar medical needs being grouped together with one medical team. As the CUSP executive on Weinberg-4C, I helped create a team structure similar to what we had in the ICU. Thanks to that work, James is one of eight patients Rich has on the unit. In this way, the nurses have more experience working with patients like James and can better identify and mitigate risks before they turn into complications. Also, this enables the entire team to make rounds together, including family members. The care plan goes into the daily goals sheet and is also written on a whiteboard in the patient's room so the patient's family and everyone can see it clearly. The nurse also identifies a patient's discharge date forty-eight hours in advance and writes the discharge date on the whiteboard. This not only clarifies the plan for everyone in the unit, but it answers the question: "What needs to happen before this patient can go home?"

James will also have the benefit of using the safe medication pumps—a CUSP initiative developed in the MICU that has spread to other units, including Weinberg-4C. If James becomes agitated for any reason and it is necessary to increase his sedation medication, the new medication pumps will automatically set his medication levels back to normal, protecting James from an accidental overdose. With this, we can treat his pain better and prevent him from being harmed.

Similarly, James will be protected from alarm fatigue. Let's say that the stresses of surgery and anesthesia have given James low blood pressure and low blood oxygen levels, making his heart beat faster in order to compensate. In the past, the nurse might have moved the upper limit of the heart monitor up so it would reduce the number of false alarms and prevent alarm fatigue. But the nurse might not have moved the lower number up as well, putting James at great risk. However, because of CUSP work (first originated in MPCU-4), James's alarm is set at a range of twenty beats per minute below and twenty beats per minute above whatever his average rate is.

James will also benefit from another CUSP initiative that came from MPCU-4, central line maintenance. This ingenious method for helping nurses effectively identify when to change the tubing that connects to James's central line, will help prevent a serious infection risk.

This kind of cross-fertilization was relatively rare in U.S. hospitals, including Hopkins, prior to CUSP. Now it is common. When something is successful in one unit, it often quickly spreads to other units in the hospital, usually by eager CUSP champions like Melinda Sawyer, who helped develop the system for central line maintenance when she was nurse manager on MPCU-4. Melinda literally walked around to other units in the hospital and told them about her idea and how well it had worked.

"Nobody was paying me to do this, or telling me to do this. I was just so excited about this new procedure I wanted to tell other units about it," she told me at the time.

Indeed, one of the goals of CUSP is to create a learning community throughout the organization. Prior to CUSP it was exceedingly hard to share good ideas from one unit to another. With CUSP, there is a safety team on each unit, a team that understands the science of safety, and we can connect those teams in a variety of ways to foster safety and learning. For example, to improve care of cardiac surgical patients, we can link preoperative, OR, ICU, and floor CUSP teams to design handoff tools. Or we can link all the ICUs to address a common ICU problem. With CUSP we have the wiring in place that permits us to share knowledge throughout the institution.

James is also safer in Weinberg-4C thanks to the presence of nurse practitioners and wireless monitors. If James is in danger, a unit-based nurse practitioner will be by his side in less than a minute. In the past a nurse would have had to respond to an alarm and page a surgeon, who might have been in the operating room or otherwise unavailable or hard to reach. Meanwhile the patient's condition could continue to deteriorate. Sometimes it would be too late by the time the call was answered. Luckily with the initiatives we enacted, that seldom happens now.

James has survived his surgery, recovered well, and is ready to be discharged. Once again, medication reconciliation will ensure that James has all the necessary medications registered with the pharmacy before he leaves, so he will carry the right medications home with him. The family will have been notified forty-eight hours prior to discharge so everyone can adjust his or her schedule accordingly and the patient can make a pleasant and easy transition home. In addition, the hospital team communicates with the home health nurse and the patient's primary care physician to ensure they know James's in-hospital treatments and his care plan after discharge. Similarly, the home health team members report any complications they identify back to Rich and the entire care team. This ensures we learn from our mistakes, many of which are identified after hospital discharge.

Thanks to CUSP work in the radiation oncology department, James's outpatient experience after being discharged has also improved. This team was born out of an adverse event—they provided the wrong radiation treatment to a patient. However, instead of just recovering from the incident, forgetting about it, and moving on, the staff decided to try to learn from it. They formed a CUSP team, conducted a detailed analysis of their safety process, identified and reduced risks, and even published their results.

Today this department has one of the best safety records at

Hopkins. Before James leaves the hospital, the radiation therapist starts a series of weekly meetings with Dr. Joseph Herman, the oncologist in charge of James's care. Joseph and the team coordinate James's radiation treatment regimen with his chemotherapy schedule. That way James, who lives an hour away from Hopkins, only has to come once a week to get his treatments, instead of the normal schedule, which is twice a week. The team also schedules James for his radiation simulation session while he is still an inpatient. In this session they make a foam mold of his body so that the oncologist can be sure James doesn't move during treatments, making the radiation more accurate and more effective. This improved communication between teams ensures that James's radiation sessions start on time.

In the past a doctor would recommend radiation but often that message would not reach radiation oncology and so the patient's treatments would not be scheduled, nor would he have had his simulation session. The person would drive all the way to Hopkins only to be sent home, not only wasting a trip, but delaying his treatments. These kinds of communication errors waste time and money for both patients and the hospital, and they compromise the effectiveness of the cancer treatment.

Improving communication was one of the keys that really helped improve safety on the unit, says Ruth Bell, a charge nurse on the unit. The entire staff attended a team-building seminar where the focus was on good communication. After that seminar, the team had posters placed throughout the unit to remind clinicians to keep communication open. "Now everyone knows each patient's care plan and what role each of us plays in that plan," says Ruth.

This unit also started its own hand-washing initiative to complement the work begin done hospitalwide. This helps to better ensure that along with his other health concerns, James does not also contract a hospital-acquired infection on one of his outpatient visits.

In addition, James will be given a gown to wear when he gets his radiation. In the past, patients would be treated in their street clothes. But tight belts and other clothing pull on skin, making the target area for the radiation inaccurate. With gowns, the treatments are more precise and more effective.

Last but not least, the staff had a problem keeping wheelchairs in the unit. Most of the wheelchairs would end up in the parking lot. The CUSP team talked to maintenance and had the wheelchairs labeled so it was clear which chairs belonged to the oncology unit. They also asked the maintenance crew to routinely scan the parking lot and return any missing wheelchairs back to the unit.

For our second hypothetical case, we look at a completely different part of the hospital, the Department of Psychiatry. This time our imaginary patient is a twenty-three-year-old white female, Nancy. One night the police respond to a report of a disturbance in downtown Baltimore. When they arrive they find Nancy at a bus stop, partially undressed. A crowd has gathered and she is screaming at them and gesticulating wildly. When the police try to talk to her, she swears at them, babbles unintelligibly, and gets violent. Suspecting drugs, alcohol, or mental illness, the police take her into custody and deliver her to the Johns Hopkins psychiatric emergency department (psych ED).

Psychiatry has its own emergency department contained within the general emergency department (ED). The director of the unit, Dr. Patrick Triplett, and his team have done a lot to improve safety in this unit. This is an excellent example of how CUSP has both directly and indirectly helped a unit improve. Much of the work here came out of these clinicians' desire to make things better and some of it was independent of CUSP. Yet Patrick will tell you that the CUSP work helped train clinicians to identify problems and gave them the confidence and tools to fix many of these problems. It also helped gain hospitalwide support for these initiatives. Finally CUSP did a lot to improve communication and teamwork, which is the backbone of patient safety.

One of the safety efforts led by Patrick and his team was to improve communication with police, which makes Nancy's handoff to Hopkins much more effective. Patrick helped the city develop a curriculum to train police officers on how to work better with psychiatric centers like Hopkins. As part of that training they taught police how to better document behaviors and other details of an arrest that might help doctors diagnose the patient. Just as with any disease, the more information they have on a patient's medical condition, the more success the staff has in treating a problem. Furthermore, this information might help doctors better assess whether Nancy is a threat to herself, other patients, or staff in the ED.

Thanks to this training, the doctors learn Nancy is violent (she resisted arrest) and is potentially a suicide risk (she got very depressed after being apprehended and talked about how nobody cared whether she lived or died). Everything in their report goes into our files—where she was picked up, family contacts, and where she lives. If Nancy is in psychiatric distress she might not be able to supply this information accurately, so the doctors rely heavily on the police report. Also, if Nancy needs to be admitted against her will, this report from the officers can be used in that petition. This improved communication goes both ways. If the hospital decides Nancy is fine and releases her, they will notify the officers.

A small, crowded space, the psych ED has seven beds and two

isolation rooms. Since psych ED is contained in the general ED, there has traditionally been tension between medical and psychiatric staff. This often happens between departments, but given the stress inherent to emergencies and the tight quarters in the psych ED, conflicts between the two departments and the associated miscommunications create serious risks to patients.

In Nancy's struggle with the police, she got a sizable cut on her forehead. This cut requires medical attention, which means the two departments have to coordinate care. Having a full-time director to oversee the psych ED has done wonders to help the teams work better together. Before Patrick took over, a rotating team of psychiatrists handled this responsibility, and their presence in the ED was unreliable. Now the medical staff has a regular face they see all the time. Patrick has developed strong relationships with the attending physicians from the emergency department and meets with them regularly. The two departments also have members on each other's CUSP teams; this has greatly improved both culture and communication.

Thanks to this improved relationship, the two teams work together and decide that Nancy needs medical care first. To facilitate a handoff like this, the team created a form that clarifies the patient's overall care plan. The form is essentially a checklist that ensures the patient is safe at all times. It reads as follows:

❏ When the patient's medical problems are resolved send him or her back to the psych ED.
❏ When the patient's medical problems are resolved he or she can be released.
❏ The patient is an elopement risk.
❏ The patient has a history of violence.

Thanks to this handoff checklist, while Nancy's head wound is being treated she will be monitored to ensure she does not harm herself or others in the general ED. The medical team will also know not to release her, but to return her to the psych ED.

Better communication between these two teams is critical to patient safety. Many conditions that would appear to be psychiatric are in fact medical. Patrick says they once had a case where a person was picked up driving down Orleans Street completely naked with all his doors open. It turned out he was not mentally ill, nor intoxicated. This patient had a severe infection and was so hot and confused he took off his clothes and opened his car doors to cool off. To catch these anomalies, the care team does a basic medical screening and head CT scan right away to try to diagnose the problem. The psychiatric staff needs to have a good relationship with the medical staff to get these tests done quickly.

The psych ED also introduced trained psychiatric nurses to the unit; previously it had depended on general ED nurses. This helped with communication both inside the unit and between the psych ED and psychiatric floor units. Not only are these nurses trained to handle psychiatric cases but they speak the same technical language as the other members of the psychiatry department. This creates continuity throughout Nancy's care. Since she is always in contact with trained staff, she is under constant professional psychiatric supervision, making handoffs efficient and accurate. Any new information regarding her behavior will be properly notated and added to her file.

The psych ED improved the way it trains and supervises staff in both the psych and general EDs—from attendings all the way down to medical students. Patrick remembers having a conversation with a medical student once who asked him if he should "take down" a psychiatric patient if the patient got violent (not a good idea). That incident sent a clear message that training was lacking.

Triage has been an ongoing problem, says Patrick, but they are making good progress thanks to the group CUSP meetings. Patients used to be searched by security for drugs and contraband at the triage station. This is a very small area and searching patients only added confusion. That has been changed. They also improved the process through which they recognize high-risk patients and get them back into the unit fast. Since Nancy came in with police, and is already considered a risk, she would be treated immediately. Furthermore, the police would be asked to leave their guns in a special lockbox before going back to the psych unit—another safety precaution that protects everyone in both EDs.

Patrick says they also discussed the physical environment in the CUSP meetings. The staff looked especially for anchoring points where a patient could potentially hang him- or herself. In Nancy's case this is significant since she has been recognized as a potential suicide risk. They identified quite a few areas of risk, including an old IV hook hanging from the ceiling. In addition, they made the sprinkler heads so they would break away and the curtains so they would tear away.

CUSP also helped the unit identify some risks associated with violent patients. In our case Nancy gets agitated and starts throwing chairs around the psych ED. In response, staff in the psych ED trip the "blue bells"—an alarm system that notifies security. A CUSP meeting revealed that this system was not wired to the main security office as previously believed, but only to the desk at the front door. CUSP helped them get the money to rewire these alarms and now they ring in the main security office as well. Now the entire security team is alerted of Nancy's outburst. They dispatch a team and the situation is controlled.

It is time for Nancy to be transported to Meyer-5, a psychiatric floor unit. The handoffs to the floor have improved significantly thanks to the addition of full-time psych nurses and to better overall communication. The psych ED resident telephones the floor attending physician and the nurses also talk. An improved handoff form goes with Nancy that contains all the information about her arrest and about her stay in the psych ED. A security guard, a nurse, and a resident go with Nancy on the transport to ensure that she is safe. When Nancy arrives on the floor the nurse stays until the patient is properly settled into the unit.

Once Nancy is on the floor, she will similarly benefit from what nurse manager Terry Goodwyn and her team have done to make that unit safer. One of the first things they did was to make the unit suicideproof. In the bathrooms they had the plumbing placed inside the walls so there is no place to anchor anything that might be used for hanging. They also had all the closet hooks rated for fifty pounds maximum weight. The chains on the blinds are breakaway, as are the automatic sprinkler heads in the ceiling. Anything and everything that Nancy could possibly use to do herself harm was removed or modified.

Terry says they also had problems with falls: "We had as many as twenty falls per week." Terry recognizes that her patients are a fall risk for many reasons: because of neurological problems related to trauma or to a disease like Alzheimer's or Parkinson's, or simply because their medication makes them drowsy or affects their motor skills. As part of her treatment Nancy is on benzodiazepine, which makes her light-headed and a fall risk.

In order to make their patients safer the team identified areas in the unit that would increase their risk of fall and injury. It was discovered that the chairs were low and hard to get in and out of; the same was true with toilet seats. Also the shower had a very smooth floor that the housekeeping staff kept waxed—add water to that, and you have a serious fall issue. So they replaced the chairs, fixed the toilet seats, and had the floors redone so they had a rough surface.

Just like Patrick Triplett's work, much of the work done on the psychiatric floor units was not directly the result of CUSP. Much of the safety improvements that occurred in these units came about due to the hard work of safety-minded clinicians. However, CUSP clearly enhanced this work by improving teamwork and communication, garnering support from the administration and making safety a science. For example CUSP improved the way nurses interacted with their managers. Today they are much more comfortable coming to Terry with their problems or concerns. CUSP gave them the assurance that they would be listened to, not penalized. CUSP also continues to provide a framework for additional defects to be discovered and corrected.

Our third example involves one of the most common diseases we see at Hopkins: heart failure. An overweight fifty-five-year-old woman named Ethel is found in bed by her husband—she won't wake up or talk to him. When he finally gets her to respond, she is speaking incoherently. Her husband calls 911, an ambulance arrives, and the medics begin treating Ethel. She has the classic signs of heart failure: she has a heart rate of 130, blood pressure of 90 over 49, and she is breathing 35 times a minute; she also has a slight fever of 99.8 degrees. The EMTs take her to the Johns Hopkins emergency department.

In the past, a triage nurse examining Ethel might have missed that she was experiencing heart failure. Now all patients coming into the ED are also seen by a doctor. This way the hospital is more likely to catch cases that need immediate attention. The doctor instantly sees that Ethel is at great risk and she is admitted. Ethel collapses, so they bring her into the critical care bay and a team of nurses, technicians, physicians, and residents resuscitate her.

"The teamwork in this emergency environment has improved significantly thanks to Peter's safety culture teamwork," says Dr. Julius Cuong Pham, an attending physician in the ED. Julius says staff had a lack of clarity in terms of responsibilities and a lack of familiarity each other's roles. "Participating in CUSP, watching the science of safety videos, bringing experts in to talk to staff, and discussing difficult problems helped physicians and nurses improve teamwork significantly."

After the clinicians resuscitate Ethel, they decide to place a central line, so they use their central line kit and the checklist. They also discover Ethel has pneumonia. Thanks to a CUSP initiative, the diagnosis and treatment of this pneumonia have been accelerated. In the old days the doctor would have had to remember to keep checking with radiology to see if the chest X-ray had revealed pneumonia; today the radiologist will call as soon as he or she spots it. They also keep the necessary antibiotics for pneumonia in the ED so they can administer them immediately. Before, this could have taken hours.

The team decides Ethel needs to be ventilated. The CUSP team has created a time-out for this procedure to make sure they have all the right equipment and that the respiratory therapist, the nurse, and the physician are all ready to go. If an intubation goes wrong— let's say the team does not correctly insert the breathing tube into the patient's windpipe—the patient can die. Thanks to CUSP, Ethel is protected from this life-threatening error with their intubation checklist. The intubation goes flawlessly. Now she is ready to go to the Osler-4 unit.

One of the most important initiatives Hopkins has taken that will drastically improve Ethel's care is that it introduced a heart failure care coordinator. Assistant director of medical nursing Joanne Ioannou helped develop the initiative. Joanne, a former nurse manager on Osler-4, was very involved in CUSP in the early years when it was first introduced on that unit. What CUSP taught her has never left her.

"You saw the magic, that it worked and made sense," Joanne says, "then you did your own work. That's what happened with my initiative to improve heart failure care. I started this task force when I was still a nurse manager on Osler-4. CUSP inspired me to think of inpatient programs to help transition patients while they are in the hospital to understand their diagnosis, what is going on with them and their disease, how to manage signs and symptoms to be a part of their care."

Joanne's work is just another example of how CUSP not only helps safety leaders identify and eliminate risk in a unit, but it also indirectly supports safety initiatives that are independent of CUSP. Joanne's improvements to heart failure care did not come out of a CUSP meeting or a CUSP team. Instead it was inspired by the success she had experienced with CUSP teams in Osler-4. She learned that if you wanted to change something you could do it. She saw that Hopkins supported this work and it gave her the confidence to go out on her own. Our goal here is patient safety. How that goal is achieved, or who gets the credit, is not important. What is important is that we achieve measurable improvements in safety.

Heart failure has one of the highest readmission rates. These readmissions are costly and often associated with complications. Joanne believes this is due in large part to the fact that patients typically do not understand the reasoning behind all the medications they are taking or the strict diet they are supposed to be on. Reducing ambiguity applies not only to doctors and nurses communicating but also to communicating with patients. If patients are unclear about their care plan, if instructions are ambiguous, they will likely make mistakes.

Dietary regimes are extremely restrictive for heart failure patients. Heart disease is a condition where the heart expands and cannot pump blood efficiently. When a person gains a lot of fluid weight this inefficiency drops to a critical point. The patient gets short of breath and starts to lose various functions and must be admitted to the hospital. If treatment succeeds in getting the fluid level down, symptoms go away and the patient is released. Unfortunately, once a person has an episode of heart failure he or she most likely will always be in danger of it. Yet these patients often go back to old habits of eating high-sodium foods like hot dogs and potato chips. This kind of diet inevitably results in fluid gain and the patient returns to the hospital with the same symptoms. It's a revolving door. In order to stop this revolving door from continuing to put these patients in danger, Joanne and her team knew that they needed somebody on the inpatient side to teach these concepts to patients so they could better understand the disease. It keeps them safer and keeps them out of the hospital. The same could be said about diabetes, depression, lung disease, and a host of other ailments that have exceedingly complicated care plans. Without clear instructions, mistakes will occur.

"Care coordinators help teach the patient what they need to know about their disease and their meds—these patients go home with a ton of medication," says Joanne.

In Ethel's case, as soon as she is admitted she is assigned a care coordinator who begins educating her on how to better manage her health so she will not keep returning to the hospital or, worse yet, suffer total cardiac arrest and possibly die. Similarly, the coordinator makes sure that Ethel understands the purpose behind the medications she is on, as well as how much medicine she is supposed to take and how frequently. It's like having a personal trainer. The care coordinator works with Ethel the entire time she is in the hospital, using an array of teaching tools and repeatedly quizzing Ethel to make sure these lessons are taking hold. By asking patients to repeat everything they have learned, the patients come to own the lessons. If a clinician just tells a patient to do something, the patient often views it as the clinician's responsibility and doesn't stick to the regime. Moreover, patients often interpret instructions differently from how the clinician intended them. For example, when we instruct patients to take medicine twice a day, some take them at seven a.m. and noon. We intend the doses to be spaced twelve hours apart; yet our instructions do not clearly communicate this. Studies show if patients learn and then teach back, retention goes from 20 percent to 75 percent. Finally, once Ethel is discharged the care coordinator repeatedly calls her at home to see how she is doing.

Our last example is another common disease: stroke. In this case, our patient is a seventy-year-old man named George with a history of smoking and hypertension who suddenly develops weakness on one side of his body. He calls 911 and is taken to the emergency room at Hopkins. The ambulance most likely will recognize this as a stroke emergency and radio ahead. But if the ED staff hasn't been alerted, the triage team is similarly trained to identify stroke victims and will immediately notify the brain attack team. This is a newly formed group of highly skilled physicians whose focus is emergency stroke care; they have a response time of fifteen minutes. There is also an attending physician on call twenty-four hours a day who is no more than one hour from the hospital.

Much of the improved care George will receive was made possible by neurologist Eric Aldrich, who cares for patients on the stroke unit. He has spent most of his career at Hopkins working to establish a comprehensive stroke program. In fact, it was his work that created the brain attack team.

"Before brain attack teams were introduced, many hospitals would assume there was nothing they could do for patients except give them an aspirin, sit them in the corner, and hope they got better. If the patients survive they would be shipped off to rehab," Eric says.

In an ischemic stroke (stroke due to a blood clot) it is essential that you deliver tissue plasminogen activator (tPA) as soon as possible. TPA dissolves the clot that is blocking the artery and restores blood flow to the brain, preventing further damage and resulting neurological deficits. Every second of delay results in the loss of brain cells and a greater chance that the patient will die. Getting tPA fast can mean the difference between having no long-term limitations and being paralyzed in half of your body—unable to eat, drink, or talk. To improve this time-to-tPA, the brain attack team purchased more sophisticated pagers. Before these new pagers were introduced, when the ED staff paged the neurology department for a consult they would have to add 911 to the end of the return number to indicate it was a stroke emergency. The ED staff would then wait for a callback. Some people were forgetting to type in the 911, and as result, the neurology resident would not see it as a stroke emergency. If the neurologist on duty was already doing a consult, and didn't recognize it as an emergency, she would wait until she was finished before responding to the page, losing precious time.

The new pagers go directly to the brain attack team. They also have a drop-down menu that allows the ED to put in more information, so there is no confusion as to whether it is a stroke and the team can get in motion immediately.

The ED has also been trained to treat strokes as they would an emergency trauma. Because the hospital requires that a patient give his name to receive care, trauma patients are sometimes provided an alias to get things moving. This was extended to include stroke patients.

The next thing for George is to give him a priority CT scan to see if his stroke is ischemic or hemorrhagic (due to bleeding). If it is a clot and the team could determine that the stroke happened within three hours, they would give George tPA. After three hours tPA is not recommended. Similarly, if the stroke is hemorrhagic they will not give tPA—if the hemorrhage is large, they will consult neurosurgery. All of this now happens within thirty minutes, most of the time within ten.

After George is treated in the ED he goes either to a floor or to the neurosciences ICU (NCCU). In our case, his stroke is hemorrhagic but does not require immediate surgery, so they send him to the NCCU.

Thanks to Eric's work, George's testing regime is already in motion before he even hits the NCCU. Neurology now demands a near-immediate turnaround on these tests. Time is of the essence with stroke patients. Studies have shown that the sooner you can administer the correct treatments to stroke patients the better chance they have at recovering function. In the past they could have waited days for these results.

Eric's work is an excellent example of standardizing care and the benefits of doing so. A hospital like Johns Hopkins treats patients with thousands of different diagnoses and procedures. For some of these, we do not know enough to standardize—the evidence is immature and we need to depend on intuition and experience. For other diseases for which we have a lot of knowledge, like stroke, patient outcomes greatly improve with standardization. Yet it takes a scientist like Eric to know which processes need standardization, to overcome barriers to getting patients treated quickly, to measure results, and to change the system so all patients get the best care.

In the NCCU George gets a central line. Thanks to CUSP team executive Ed Miller, this procedure has been even further improved to ensure that George receives the proper procedure and precautions. The NCCU linked their central line cart to the system that orders medication for the unit. Now when they use items out of the cart, the items are automatically replaced.

The nurses also start educating George so he will know how to recognize the signs if he starts experiencing another stroke. He will also learn how to change his lifestyle to prevent this from happening again. They will talk to him about quitting smoking, changing his diet, and managing his medications, giving him a better understanding of each.

When George leaves this unit he goes to the Meyer-9 stroke unit. CUSP also helped the NCCU team improve its handoffs to this unit. The NCCU staff actually went to the Meyer-9 and Meyer-8 (the two units that work with the NCCU most) and asked those nurses and doctors what they wanted included in the handoff. As NCCU clinical nurse specialist Betsy Zink says, "The handoff was much more for them than it was for us, so we listened to what they needed and modeled our handoff according to what Meyer-8 and Meyer-9 wanted."

She explains that they added stroke-specific things, for example, how much IV antihypertensive medicine the patient received in the last twenty-four hours, as well as when the last dose was given and how often the patient was receiving the drug. The nurses and doctors in the Meyer units also need to know if the patient has been given a swallow screen (a test that indicates whether the person has lost the ability to swallow—essential knowledge the unit needs so they can adjust the patient's care to prevent aspiration pneumonia from developing).

In the stroke unit on Meyer-9 (also known as the brain recovery unit) they have a dedicated stroke team that cares for these patients. In the old days these patients might have been scattered around the hospital. Now all stroke victims are placed in the same unit, which means teams can make rounds together. Just like in the ICU or Rich's service on Weinberg-4C, these patients are surrounded by a unified dedicated team of specialists, all of whom are highly trained and experienced in caring for stroke victims. Because they have most of their patients in one area, both of the attending physicians on the stroke team have offices adjacent to the unit.

After George is stable he will leave Meyer-9 and go to rehab on Halsted-3. Halsted-3 has a dedicated CUSP team and its nurse manager, Sue Verrillo, is a huge fan of the way CUSP has improved communication on her unit. "Lack of communication was our biggest problem; we have so many teams working here, it is often hard to get everyone on the same page."

To remedy this problem they developed a single electronic care plan sheet that will document every aspect of George's treatment. Each sheet has a drop-down menu and there are also spaces to write notes. Fall risk, deep vein thrombosis prophylaxis, pain status, nursing care plan—all of this goes in one place and on one shared drive and everyone writes on it every shift.

In addition, this unit modified the daily goals to fit the needs of the unit. Since they have such a large number of care teams, group rounding was not always possible. So the staff meets daily with all the teams so everyone can better understand the care plan for George. Everything that is discussed in the meeting is documented on his chart.

The team also keeps an electronic notebook that includes patient history, what was talked about at team meetings, family goals, as well as discharge planning. They use this notebook to determine when George is ready to go home and to assist him with that transition. In addition, they have reviewed all the educational materials being given to the patients on the various stroke floors to make sure George is getting the same message throughout the hospital.

When George is through with his care and on his way home, he will understand clearly how to recognize and avoid another stroke and also what each of his medications does and why they are important. The physicians also communicate with his primary care physician regarding what treatments George received in the hospital, what the outpatient care plan is, and what George should do for follow-up care.

One of the best things Sue says came out of CUSP is that they do not allow bad communication to happen. "We try to have the entire team—physical therapy, occupational therapy, speech nursing, physicians, social workers, home health, and pharmacy—everyone at the table. It is truly multidisciplinary. We encourage an open culture where we call each other on anything related to patient safety. Nothing falls through the cracks. If a doctor puts the orders in wrong we nail him on it. Today I nailed the medical director for sending a patient to the floor without the proper paperwork."

Just as is true with the advances in patient safety in treating cancer, mental illness, heart disease and countless other conditions, some of the safety initiatives associated with stroke care came directly out of CUSP, some were indirectly influenced by CUSP, and some were helped along simply because safety awareness at Hopkins was on the rise.

When Eric Aldrich first started building his stroke center back in the late 1990s, CUSP was in its infancy. On his own initiative, Eric approached senior executives about getting money for a stroke program, but budgets were tight. Undaunted, he got a ten-thousand-dollar educational grant, found some empty rooms on Meyer-7, grabbed some used black-and-white heart monitors out of the basement and mounted them on plywood, and created a four-bed dedicated stroke unit.

In 2004, after CUSP had begun to spread through Hopkins, he met with executives Rich Grossi and Ed Miller, and this time he got what he needed. Ed Miller literally said a stroke center at Hopkins was a "no-brainer," according to Eric. Today Hopkins has a six-bed brain rescue unit housed on Meyer-9, staffed by eight fully trained neurology nurses, a full-time nurse coordinator, and two attending physicians. Eric took his makeshift four-bed unit and turned it into a certified stroke center that has since become the best center in the Mid-Atlantic region and one of the best in the country.

"This CUSP work created an environment that patient safety is important, and all of a sudden all these programs were receiving funding that they may not have gotten before," says Eric. "Put it this way: it didn't hurt that Ed Miller was on the CUSP team in the NCCU when we approached him for funding. This heightened safety awareness raised the water level and multiple boats were floated. Safety programs which might have struggled or withered on the vine prosper in this environment. When you get executives on the floor, then it becomes real. The general has a better sense of where to send the ammo. The best things you can do to get people motivated are create a fertile environment and get the hell out of the way. That's what this work did. It created a fertile environment for patient safety. Now when I plant seeds they are not landing on pavement."

And the win-win here is that Eric's work not only made things safer for patients like George, it also turned stroke from being a loss leader into a department that pays its own bills. The rising tide of patient safety awareness is a tide I have risen on as well. The Institute of Medicine report and the work done by the Institute for Healthcare Improvement, the Joint Commission, and the National Quality Forum all set the stage for a national and international movement that is now taking off. We believe our biggest contribution to this wave of safety awareness is our continued insistence on scientific methods and measurement. Without strong science how can we say we made a difference? How can we look Sorrel in the eye and say with confidence that Josie would be less likely to die?

# Conclusion

====

T en years after Josie King's death Sorrel once again returned to the hospital. We met for coffee and got caught up on each other's lives. The conversation eventually came around to our common concern, patient safety. And once again, Sorrel wanted to know if we had managed to make things better in the ten years since she lost her daughter. And for the first time I really believed I could give the answer she deserved. I looked her in the eye and said, "Yes, Hopkins is safer and you played a huge part in making that happen."

She became quiet, settled back in her chair. Her tough exterior, which I had grown to accept because of her loss, melted away and hope and curiosity twinkled in her eye. She wanted to hear how, and I wanted to tell her.

"Hopkins and the world have a long way to go. But thanks to everyone's hard work, patient safety has become a priority here and there is no turning back. There has been an explosion of new methods and interventions to improve safety, much of it inspired by our efforts at Hopkins and Michigan—efforts that we are now exporting to the country and the world."

Sorrel had an anxious smile. "And pediatrics? What are you

doing to make kids safer? Tell me what you have done that could have prevented Josie from dying."

"Thanks to the generous donation you made to the Children's Center, Marlene and her team have made enormous strides in improving safety. Every Wednesday the director of the Children's Center, George Dover, Marlene, and members of her team make safety rounds. They walk around the center, ask staff about hazards to patients, and follow through to minimize those hazards. We also have an error reporting system that all staff can access and use to report errors. Marlene and her team review these error reports, investigate them, and take action to reduce the risks. The medical students who rotate through pediatrics also learn how to investigate mistakes, as do the pediatric residents. They are producing a whole cadre of students who really understand patient safety.

"The team has made tremendous progress, especially in reducing bloodstream infections, like the one that triggered the avalanche that led to Josie's death. The Children's Center regularly trains its residents on how to resuscitate a child. When they started, errors were happening 30 percent of the time. With the training, performance has been nearly flawless. They have also made tremendous progress in improving pediatric medication safety; they have special pharmacists on the units and many more safety checks. Though I cannot say that we will never have a medication error that harms a patient, I can say these errors are dramatically reduced.

"Marlene has spread this program to sixty pediatric ICUs in the United States. They have nearly eliminated central line infections in these hospitals and she plans to spread this to all pediatric ICUs in the country, and hopefully the world. In fact, this work has grown so much that Marlene now has a division of patient safety within the Department of Pediatrics. I believe it is the first division of safety in any academic department, anywhere in the world. Traditionally departments have always had directors of training and research and clinical directors; what they need are directors of quality and safety. Today pediatrics has one in Marlene.

"The PICU team now uses daily goals and has a solid CUSP team. Communication among team members has improved markedly. The unit has computerized physician order entry and also has much more formal handoffs with the floor teams; this way no information is lost. Today they would be much more likely to identify Josie's dehydration. And since they have virtually eliminated bloodstream infections, Josie likely would never have developed the infections that triggered this dehydration.

"Since Josie's death, Marlene has developed a pediatric hospitalist program whose sole purpose is to medically comanage children under two years old who are on surgical services. We likely need hospitalists to comanage all children but at least we have them for the youngest and most vulnerable, like Josie.

"Also, nurses or parents can now summon a rapid response team—an ICU team that responds quickly to deteriorating patients. When you were concerned about Josie, you could have called one of these teams. More than likely this team would have taken action— moving Josie to the PICU and making sure she got hydrated. The same is true of the nurses or anyone on the floor who believes there is reason for concern.

"Recently I met with a senior nurse in the unit where Josie died and she told me a story that was hauntingly similar to yours. With tears in her eyes, she recounted how a child on the surgical service was deteriorating and the surgeons were not responding. The nurse called the PICU to immediately evaluate the child. The child was admitted and suffered no harm but could have if not for the nurse's actions. The nurse told me, 'I will never let another Josie King happen when I am on, never. I will carry a child to the PICU if I need to. Peter, never again.' Her determination, etched in her soul by painful memories of Josie, was palpable.

"That's not to say we don't have more work to do. Even though the addition of rapid response teams, hospitalists, and nurse practitioners have made units safer, nurses constantly tell me they are still struggling to get some surgeons to listen and respond effectively to the entire care team. In my many travels to hospitals all over the country, I hear the same complaint."

I went on to relate a story about this to Sorrel. We had recently had a problem in one of the adult ICUs that clearly illustrated both the work that lies ahead of us and the progress we have made. A resident called a surgery fellow in the middle of the night to help place a central line. He walked into the unit and put gloves on, but no cap or gown, and proceeded to place the central line. The nurses tried to stop him, but he told them to screw off. He said, "I am not doing that. This is stupid." The nurses pushed back and he pushed back more. So the nurses went and found the charge nurse and the nurse practitioner. The surgery fellow threw a big temper tantrum and a big power struggle ensued. What was even worse was that the nurses went to the attending surgeon and he did nothing. The fellow inserted the line without the precautions to prevent the patient from acquiring a central line infection. When I got paged at home, they explained the situation and I told them I would speak to the fellow in the morning.

When I met with the fellow I said, "If you want to succeed in this business, being technically good is the entry fee, but it won't make you a great physician. Being interpersonally good is what is going to help you rise to the top and improve your patient's outcomes. You have a lot to offer medicine. However, to realize your potential you will need to be both technically good and a good team player. How do you think your behavior last night was perceived by the nurses?"

He said, "Well, I suppose I was a little rough."

I said, "Rough. You acted like a jerk. What you and I need to talk about is why and what we are going to do so that won't happen again. I can't let patients be at risk and I can't have you upsetting the staff. So help me understand why you behaved that way."

He began to let his guard down and actually got tearful. He told me he had been up for three days doing transplants. The rules that prohibit physicians from working long hours don't always apply to fellowships. So he was working like a dog, sleep deprived, and likely acting like a paranoid schizophrenic. I also learned he was having marital problems. It is no wonder that when he was pushed, he exploded. It is not an excuse for his behavior but at least it helps us better understand how to prevent these kinds of scenarios from playing out. Simply disciplining physicians will not work. We clearly need to address the systems in which they practice. As part of their medical education we need to offer training on how to manage this stress. We need to balance our technical training with emotional and social training.

A number of months later I got a page from this same fellow. He had taken a faculty position at another prestigious academic medical center. In a friendly and bubbly voice he said, "Hey, Peter, remember the talk you gave me about the science of safety and leadership, about how important it was to use the checklist and improve culture and teamwork? Thanks. It has really stuck and influenced me. I am giving a talk at a morbidity and mortality conference on patient safety and I want to know if I can use some of your slides. I found some great ones on the Web. I think many of our surgeons would benefit from your approach. We are nowhere near as far along in safety here as you are and I would really like to introduce some of your concepts into our department and hospital."

If ever there was true validation of our work. If ever we could be sure that our message was being heard loud and clear, this was it. A huge smile filled my face. I felt like a proud father. The work was really making a difference; we were beginning to reshape culture.

I told him, "This is the best thing I have heard in a while. Of course you can use any slide you want. Put your name on them and make them your own." He said, "I will."

I concluded by telling Sorrel, "These successes are far from isolated. In fact, in almost every unit I visit, I hear reports about how our work or the story of Josie changed the way they view health care. It speaks to my true belief that this kind of work unlocks the good that is in all people. In medicine, that good manifests itself in the desire to deliver the best possible care to patients. When clinicians are given the tools and support they need to reach that goal, and they get constructive feedback about it, it brings great satisfaction to their work and that only improves the patient experience."

Shortly after that meeting with Sorrel I got two pieces of news that brought me back to the roots of my work. The first was that I was asked to give the commencement speech at Fairfield University, my alma mater. The second was that I learned my stepfather was dying of cancer.

My mother married her second husband, Paul, in September 2004. Three months after the wedding he was diagnosed with colon cancer. Since then Paul had been struggling with the disease. I had recently learned that he was losing the battle.

My father's death, also from cancer, was one of the motivating factors that propelled me toward pursuing medicine and patient safety as a career. The fact that I was soon to lose a second father to cancer, and that I was scheduled to return to the campus where I first learned of my father's illness, stirred up a lot of emotion and memories.

I needed to think, and the best way for me to sort out my thoughts was to run. So I put on my running shoes and headed out the door. The North Central Railroad Trail runs north from Baltimore County into Pennsylvania. It is an old railroad track that got converted to a hiking and biking trail. It runs alongside a sleepy river where the smell of honeysuckle and pine fills the air. I often run there or go for bike rides with my son, Ethan, and daughter, Emma. I knew a quick jog wouldn't do the trick so I set out for a ten-mile run. I call these my Zen runs. When I get them right, I feel no pain, time stops, and my soul quiets. In order to get to that space, I have to run at just the right speed. If I go too fast and I breathe too hard, I don't relax enough. Similarly, if I'm too slow, I don't get the endorphins flowing. I have my own little checklist for Zen runs.

Luckily on that day I got it right. As I got into the zone, I thought about how my team and I had successfully conducted the largest valid quality improvement project in Michigan, which is now being implanted across the country. We helped to elevate patient safety as a respected science; we matured that science and began saving thousands of lives and millions of dollars. We have informed practice and health policy. We partnered with WHO and are implementing the program in several countries. We have trained medical and nursing students, residents, and attending physicians in the science of safety. We have helped improve teamwork and communication between doctors and nurses and helped restore joy to the practice of medicine. It was a long list of achievements my fellow colleagues and I could certainly be proud of.

Lifting my sunglasses to wipe the sweat from my face, I felt a strange mixture of peace and anxiety. Peace that we were fortunate enough to do something that broadly helped patients, changed practice and was personally rewarding, but also anxiety about the tremendous amount of work that lay ahead and the uncertainty that came with that work.

I remember Chris Goeschel asking me what was next. I told her I couldn't say for sure. These concepts are by no means limited to health care. I recently gave a talk in London to Barclays Bank about applying our theories to finance. It was a rousing success and led me to believe that these principles are successful because they are based on universal truths about people, teams, and organizations. They are about the need to make the world better, to contribute to something bigger than ourselves, to be accountable for results yet encourage innovation, and to feel proud of our commitments and achievements. Our work in creating checklists, measuring progress toward goals, and changing culture applies not only to bloodstream infections, but to banking and finance, personal fitness and dieting, and relationships with our loved ones. It is a general model for leadership.

With sweat stinging my eyes and the sun warming my face, I also reflected on my definitions of leadership. Leadership is the ability to address problems that make the world better. It's about inviting people into the process and providing hope that they can make a change.

As I continued running, I wondered how I could share this concept with the graduates of Fairfield. I wanted to tell them about our work in patient safety and what we had accomplished and were accomplishing. But these students would be heading out into the world to face a myriad of professional and personal challenges. A talk based solely on our achievements in medicine would most likely bore them to death. I needed a way to connect our work to the challenges they would face in the coming years. As I passed a bend in the river where a mother and her daughter rode bikes together, it suddenly came to me: Josie was my connection to reality; I would make her their connection as well.

Running helps me come up with ideas, but writing helps me clarify them. I knew what I wanted to say, now I had to return to my house and put it down on paper.

The university kindly arranged to get a driver to take me from Baltimore to Fairfield. This was greatly welcomed since the five-hour ride gave me time to put the final touches on my speech and catch up with other work. I brought my son, Ethan, along and we spent the night at my brother Paul's house. Both my brothers, Paul and John, planned to come to the talk along with their children.

The next morning we drove onto campus, past the parking lot where my parents had told me about my father's cancer, the cafeteria and gym where I hung out with friends and swam, the lacrosse field, the dorms, and the library. I felt a sense of great illumination in returning to this place, where so many early impressions and experiences shaped who I am today. As I walked on stage in front of a crowd of more than fifteen thousand students, parents, alumni, and families, that feeling only intensified.

I started my speech like so many others. I thanked the university for inviting me and congratulated the graduates and their parents. I told them about my life as a student at Fairfield and how my brothers, my father, and my uncle had all graduated from the school. I talked about the challenges they would face in the coming years and how it was their duty to lead the way into the future. I explained the work I had done at Hopkins and in Michigan and how we were spreading that work across the globe. I shared with them how this had become my mission, my goal, and how I believed each of them would find a way to do their small part in making this world a better place. And then I told them about Josie.

I felt a familiar lump in my throat, the same tragic sorrow I had felt when I met the Kings at their house so many years ago and first talked about Josie with Sorrel and Tony. I had told this simple story hundreds of times in hundreds of different settings and it always touched me deeply. I was sure it would have the same effect here.

> An adorable eighteen-month-old girl, Josie King, who was hauntingly similar to my daughter, Emma, died of preventable mistakes; principal among them was a catheter infection.
>
> On the four-year anniversary of her death, her mother asked if Josie would be less likely to die today than four years ago. I started telling her all the stuff we were doing at Hopkins. She abruptly and appropriately cut me off; she did not want to know what we were doing; she wanted to know whether Josie would be less likely to die. She wanted to know whether patients were safer; she wanted results. At the time, neither I nor Hopkins nor the U.S. health system could give her an answer. I believe she deserves one. . . . Many thought we were too bold and doomed to failure. Others thought we were naive or downright nuts. There were too many obstacles; the resources were insufficient. When faced with challenges, many are blinded by obstacles and never start on the journey. Others see the endgame and the obstacles as something to be climbed or avoided. We focused on the endgame. We focused on the Josie Kings of the world.

# Acknowledgments

"Never doubt that a small group of thoughtful committed citizens can change the world, indeed, it is the only thing that ever has" —MARGARET MEADE.

We would like to thank our literary agents, Megan Thompson and Larry Kirshbaum of LJK Literary Management, for guiding, supporting, and promoting this project. We'd also like to thank our publisher, Hudson Street Press, and especially our editor, Meghan Stevenson, for having the vision to take on this project, and the diligence, insight, and patience necessary to help create and shape this story. —P. P. AND E. V.

I would like to thank my loving wife, Marlene, and my two wonderful children, Ethan and Emma, for their love and support. I would also like to thank my mother for instilling in me the desire to realize my dreams, the belief that hard work pays rewards, and the need to make the world better. I would like to thank my brothers, Paul and John, who have supported me over the years and helped shape the person I am.

At Hopkins I would like to thank my research team, the Quality and Safety Research Group, who works tirelessly to advance the science of patient safety, who is committed to making the world a better place, and without whom this work would not happen. I would also like to thank medical school Dean Ed Miller, hospital president Ron Peterson, and former university president William Brody. Without their courageous leadership none of this work would have been possible. I would like to thank John Ulatowski, the chair of the Department of Anesthesiology and Critical Care Medicine; Julie Freischlag, the chair of the Department of Surgery, and Beryl Rosenstein, the former vice president of medical affairs, whose strong support helped us implement many of our programs. I would also like to thank Joann Rodgers and Gary Stephenson of the media relations team, and Meg Garrett and Joanne Pollak of the legal team, who had the vision to understand that transparency is the best policy when it comes to learning about medical errors. In addition, I want to thank Chip Davis and the Center for Innovations in Quality Patient Care and the Hospital Safety, Quality and Risk committees, who unwaveringly supported these patient safety efforts. And I would like to thank the hard-working doctors, nurses, and administrators who helped launch our first patient safety studies, who developed new safety programs, and who, as a result, have made care safer.

Similarly, I would like to thank the thousands of hard-working clinicians and health care leaders at Michigan and around the world who had the courage to implement these programs, who had the discipline to collect robust data, and who have helped expanded this work and saved countless lives.

And I would especially like to thank Sorrell King for her courage and determination to make a stand against patient harm and help fuel a movement that truly has made hospitals safer.

Finally and most important, I would like to ask forgiveness from all the patients and their families who have suffered needlessly around the world. I believe that by working together, doctors, nurses, policy makers, administrators, insurers, and regulators can dramatically improve medicine and effectively deliver the level of quality care these patients rightfully deserve. —P. P.

I would like to thank my parents, John and Sandra Vohr, for their undying support for my writing, specifically on this project. They have generously supported all my endeavors with boundless love and enthusiasm and for that I am truly blessed.

At Johns Hopkins Medicine, thanks are due to President Ron Peterson and Dean Ed Miller for their support and help. I would also like to thank Gary Stephenson for his insights and guidance throughout this project, as well as Joann Rodgers for her skill, excellence, and high standards in science writing. Dr. Alfredo Quinones and Dr. Kay Redfield Jamison were also key sources of advice and guidance for me writing this project. Ramsey Flynn and Sue De Pasquale shared their experience and knowledge as accomplished writers. Elaine Freeman gave priceless advice and guidance, while Dalal Haldeman provided me with her support and wisdom. Linda Marcellino and Angelina Barbosa also deserve thanks for their hard work helping me write this book.

Lori Paine, Christine Goeschel, Dr. Sean Berenholtz, as well as many other clinicians and staff at Johns Hopkins took the time to share stories of how they are working to improve patient safety, which I am incredibly grateful for. This book would be incomplete without their experiences.

At Hopkins University I would also like to thank my colleagues, Pamela Sheff, Julie Reiser, Andrew Douglas, and Kristen Kelley for their support and advice, as well as Tristan Davies, Jean Mc-Garry and the rest of the Hopkins writing faculty for their skill and guidance.

Personally, I want to thank Elizabeth Leik for her undying friendship and support. Present and past family members Merritt McBrian, Ann Vohr, Wendy McBrian, Steven McBrian, Brian French, Neal, Mark, and Jill Vohr have also generously supported my writing over the years. I would like to sincerely thank Kate Crowe, writing professor at Evergreen State College, for being one of the first to realize I was a writer and for supporting my work over the years.

Barton Biggs, former editor of the *Cambodia Daily Newspaper*, gave me my first job as a journalist, and Marlene Roderick and Robin Smith, formerly of the *Bennington Banner Newspaper*, helped shape my skills. Patrick Perry at the *Saturday Evening Post*, Joe Cutts at *Ski Magazine*, and Dan D'Ambrosio formerly of *Adventure Cyclist Magazine* also supported my writing and helped me grow as a writer.

Finally I would like to thank Sorrel King for her passionate support and assistance, and express my sincere desire that this work—and this book—will help make medicine safer and more enjoyable for patients and clinicians alike. —E. V.

# Index